Alzheimer's Disease

A GUIDE FOR FAMILIES

Revised Edition

Lenore S. Powell, Ed.D.
with Katie Courtice

Addison-Wesley Publishing Company
*Reading, Massachusetts   Menlo Park, California   New York
Don Mills, Ontario   Wokingham, England   Amsterdam
Bonn   Sydney   Singapore   Tokyo   Madrid   San Juan
Paris   Seoul   Milan   Mexico City   Taipei*

Library of Congress Cataloging-in-Publication Data

Powell, Lenore S.
    Alzheimer's disease : a guide for families / Lenore S. Powell with
Katie Courtice. — Rev. ed.
      p.   cm.
    Includes bibliographical references and index.
    ISBN 0-201-63201-2
    1. Alzheimer's disease—Popular works. 2. Alzheimer's disease—
Patients—Family relationships. I. Courtice, Katie. II. Title.
RC523.P68 1992
616.8'31—dc20   92-35473
                                            CIP

The use of information from the USP DI, Volume 2 (1991), is by permission of the U.S. Pharmacopoeial Convention. © 1991 by The USP Convention, Inc.

Material adapted from Thomas Crook, Ph.D., and Samuel Gershon, M.D., *Strategies for the Development of an Effective Treatment for Senile Dementia* (1981). Published by Mark Powley Associates,
Inc., New Canaan, CT.

Some of the exercises in Chapter 16 are adapted from *How to Keep Slender and Fit after Thirty* by
Bonnie Prudden, by permission of the author. Copyright © 1961, 1969 by Bonnie Prudden.

Cover design by Lynne Reed
Text design by Janis Owens
Set in 11-point Janson by Shepard Poorman Communications Corp., Indianapolis, IN

5 6 7 8 9-MA-0099989796
Fifth printing, June 1996

This book is dedicated to my deceased parents, Dora and Israel Powell, in gratitude for their love, and to all caregivers who have the courage to face the burden of love.
—LENORE S. POWELL

To my late grandmothers, Katherine Mayes Walther and Florence North Courtice, who gave me my earliest understanding of the dignity and the difficulty of growing old.
—KATIE COURTICE

Contents

PART TWO

Understanding and Dealing with the Patient's Problems

PART THREE

Take Care of Yourself

Introduction
to the Revised Edition

Alzheimer's disease affects more than four million people in North America, but when this book was first published in 1983, few people knew that. Since then public awareness of Alzheimer's has grown dramatically through news reports, magazine articles, and television dramas such as the movie *Do You Remember Love?* starring Joanne Woodward and Richard Kiley (a show that suggested this book for further reading). By presidential proclamation November is National Alzheimer's Disease Month in the United States. This attention has prompted new services for patients and their families and increased funding for scientific research.

All of these promising developments are reflected in this new, expanded edition of *Alzheimer's Disease: A Guide for Families*, the first since 1986. We describe the most up-to-date findings on the causes of the disease, as well as the latest information on nursing homes, day care, legal matters, and other resources for caregivers. A new chapter helps caregivers deal with their fears, especially the anxiety that later in life they may develop Alzheimer's disease themselves.

We would like to take this opportunity to thank the many readers who have written to express their gratitude and appreciation for this book. People have written from all over the world to tell us how helpful it is to have someone understand their problems and how important it is to find such useful information. The reaction of these readers has been deeply moving. Perhaps one of the most rewarding aspects of writing this book is to hear that we've made a contribution both to the work of professionals who have gained insight from the book and to the lives of caregivers who have utilized it more personally. We welcome comments and letters from all readers so that we can continue to keep this book as helpful and vital as possible.

Preface

Most of the victims of Alzheimer's disease will never read this book; those who do will probably not remember or absorb much because of their failing memory.

An illness that is increasing in large proportions as our elderly population expands, Alzheimer's disease is the fourth leading cause of death. Despite this alarming statistic, in hundreds of communities throughout the nation, physicians and families alike are bewildered by the behavior of the memory-impaired person with Alzheimer's disease. Those who become the caregivers have a difficult time managing their patients at home. Feelings about themselves and their situations range from upset to anger, guilt to fear of what the future holds. The loving husbands, wives, children, siblings, cousins, in-laws, and life-long friends who watch their family members decline daily are victims also. These are the people for whom this book is written, but professionals will also benefit from its contents.

Alzheimer's Disease: A Guide for Families covers the most current researched knowledge available and medical facts about Alzheimer's disease. Symptoms, behavioral changes, and diagnostic procedures are discussed. First-hand experiences of families who have received psychotherapeutic counseling are described in an effort to provide a supportive frame of reference to the caregivers who will be reading this book.

In an attempt to help caregivers to come to terms with attitudes and feelings of helplessness, shame, frustration, fear, loneliness, and hopelessness, practical solutions to everyday problems are offered. The dilemma of placing a relative in a nursing home is dealt with frankly, and *advice* is given to the caregiver about *how* to keep himself mentally and physically in good health.

Psychologists tell us that people need each other to soothe the hurtful pain of disappointment. We also need each other for social stimulation, for competition, and to add excitement to our daily lives. When we give each other attention, we identify with each other, we sympathize with each other, and we recognize the individuality of other people. Giving and receiving praise, rewarding successful accomplishments, evaluating our opinions and abilities vis-à-vis others, and sharing our feelings are also reasons that we need each other. But mostly, people need other people to give and to receive tender sentiments and compassionate comfort and to share the joys as well as the burdens of love.

Acknowledgments

We extend special appreciation to Dr. Steven Ferris of New York University Medical Center, whose expertise was invaluable in writing the more technical aspects of this book.

To Hy Levine, Thelma Gold, and Gail Manna, whose comments on the manuscript were insightful.

To Dr. Shirley Panken, whose encouragement has sustained this project throughout.

To Amy Hymes, whose typing skills and clarity of mind were valuable assets during the entire writing of the manuscript.

To Pamela Rafford, who assisted in the painstaking transcribing of material.

To Heather Wilson, for her concise and helpful editorial comments.

To Dorothy Brunner, for her diligent research efforts.

To Lawrence M. Honig, Esq., who supplied important legal information and thoughtful discussions.

To my dear friend Dr. Marcella B. Weiner, who is a true role model—thanks for her valuable suggestions.

To John Bell, the editor of this edition, for his consistently helpful suggestions; and to Beth Burleigh, for ably supervising the production process.

To the caregivers whose individual courage and devotion in the face of personal tragedy provided the inspiration for this book.

—LENORE S. POWELL

There is no adequate way to thank my husband, Peter Basquin, for his kindness, wisdom, patience, thoughtfulness, interest, support, and love.

He was an unending source of strength during the many months of work on this book, and without his encouragement I doubt I would yet have completed it.

Many others also contributed, directly or indirectly, to the finished product. Thanks are due to our editors, Doe Coover and Elinor Neville, both for their patience and warm encouragement and also for the perceptive and creative way they helped shape and clarify the material. Sallie Gouverneur earned my eternal gratitude for her endless patience, warm, positive cheer, and reassurance whenever the material seemed about to overwhelm me.

Each person who helped in the gathering and ordering of the material in this book gave something different—some read portions of the manuscript, others offered advice or personal anecdotes and the wisdom of their own experiences, still others provided the warm and encouraging environment that makes working possible, and some did all of that and more. To each, my warm and grateful thanks, especially to my parents, Richard N. and Janet Walther Courtice, and to the other friends whose expertise, experience, and encouragement inform this book: Rev. William and Margaret Hall Cole; Mary Lou DiPietro; Harry and Esther Merrick Duncan; Mary and Becky Hardin; Glen and Sandra M. Holt; Lewis and Adria Kaplan and Deborah Frances Kaplan; Stephen C. Rector, M.D.; Ed and Toni Stern; and Nancy Shemansky.

—KATIE COURTICE

Note to Readers:

We are using the generic *he* to imply both male and female. We use the word *senile* not derogatively but as it is used popularly as a synonym for senile dementia, organic brain syndrome, memory-impaired, chronic brain syndrome, and Alzheimer's disease.

PART ONE

The Burden of Love

The burden of love is living with the helpless and knowing we cannot spare them the pain of losing themselves; nor can we spare ourselves the pain of our own losses.

CHAPTER 1

Introduction

*W*hen Lillian and Jim arrived at the school lecture hall, people were assembling for the guest speaker's travel lecture.

Jim took an aisle seat and settled Lillian next to him. Barely a minute later, she stood up and announced that it was time to leave.

"Not yet, not yet," her husband whispered quietly to her as he pulled her back down into her chair. Lillian sat, but began to rock rhythmically back and forth. The chair creaked and people began to stare. Jim tried to stop her from swaying, but she angrily twisted her arm away and stood up.

"Let's go!" she declared, loudly enough to interrupt the lecturer and make several people stare at them. Embarrassed, Jim pulled her back into her seat. "Here," he hissed, "hold your purse and sit still."

She fingered the purse aimlessly for a minute, then opened the clasp and took out a tissue, which she shredded into little ribbons. She turned to the stranger on her left and held up the tattered remains. "Look!" she said to him. "Pretty!"

Jim snatched the paper from her hand and in an aggravated tone said, "Can't you just sit still?" Lillian was quiet for a short while, perhaps as long as two minutes. Then she began to rock again, forward and back, farther and farther, until her face touched her knees and her hand reached her shoe. She pulled off her loafer and put it in her lap. She tilted it, turned it upside down, tried to put it on the wrong foot over her other shoe, and banged it on the chair in front of her.

Jim grabbed the shoe, but Lillian didn't want to let it go. They jerked the shoe back and forth in front of them until Jim, who was still stronger, managed to break her grip. He bent to hide the shoe under his chair, and as he did, Lillian jumped up and headed for the door, shouting, "I'm leaving!" Red-faced and disheveled, holding Lillian's shoe and dragging both coats behind him, Jim ran after his wife.

It's not surprising that Jim and Lillian don't go out very often. Jim finds it humiliating to receive the angry glances and hear the whispered comments. Although he becomes worn out and frustrated when Lillian does the same things at home, somehow Jim finds her behavior easier to deal with then when they are alone and she can't embarrass him. He misses the companionship of their old friends. It makes him sad to see the woman he loves behaving so strangely and to hear people refer to her as "that senile old lady."

Lillian's embarrassing behavior is a consequence of Alzheimer's disease, one of a group of illnesses in which the major symptom is loss of recent memory. It is a disease that is reaching epidemic proportions in the United States.

Her bizarre behavior, inability to reason, and memory loss result from profound changes that are taking place in her brain.

Most older people will never experience what has befallen Lillian; but the dread of senility with increasing age is a fear that even younger people harbor.

Generations of young and old alike associate mental and physical deterioration with growing older. When elderly people begin to lose even the slightest increments in hearing, vision, taste, touch, or smell, if they have some difficulty with motor skills or dexterity, or if they become somewhat fragile of limb, we immediately fear they will soon lose touch with reality. Erroneously, we conclude that irascibility, a depressed mood, unpredictable behavior, and memory lapses are the normal shortcomings of aging. When our favorite elderly aunt behaves in a childlike but charming manner, we suspect her of being in her "dotage," and when Grandpa goes into a tirade about something inconsequential, we say he's losing his marbles. What can we do but feel exasperated and put up with this odd behavior?

Although (considering the alternative) we all wish to become older, our culture conditions us to be ageist—prejudiced against older people. Despite the fact that people are living longer today than at any point in our history, instead of recognizing that there are normal changes that occur when we get older, we keep the stereotyped notion of aging as a disease. Thus it is no wonder that we fear aging as impending infirmity. Some biological deficiencies *do* occur as we age, but there is *no significant* memory impairment or intellectual deterioration in the natural developmental process of growing older that cannot be compensated for.

When an older person loses his ability to remember, think, and reason, he is suffering from *senile dementia,* a group of diseases among which Alzheimer's is probably the most insidious and most prevalent. Severe loss of these intellectual functions interferes with a person's daily functioning and may cause him to behave peculiarly and show impaired judgment. *Senile* simply means "related to old age," but it too commonly implies "weak in mind and body." Widespread use of the term *senility* reinforces the public image of elderly people as absent-minded, feeble, forgetful, and confused. People have been ashamed of admitting that a relative has a form of senile dementia—as if developing the illness were that person's own fault.

Recent-memory loss is not an inevitable fact of later life—it is a symptom of an illness. While progressive memory disability occurs in people with dementing illnesses, the loss of memory may also occur temporarily in any person in response to stress, as a reaction to medications, or as the result of fever, delirium, anxiety, or depression. Anyone who is confused or suspects that his memory is not as reliable as in the past should consider having his memory tested by a psychologist.

A person with suspected memory loss should not be satisfied with the cliché: "After all, what do you expect at your age, anyway?" We should expect and assume, as a matter of course, that as we age we will continue to be intellectually vigorous and retain the ability to learn, to think, and to remember. Any indication of memory loss requires a thorough investigation of its possible causes.

Loss of recent memory is not confined to the elderly and can stem from a variety of causes in people of any age. The depressed person, for example, whether young or old, may have memory difficulties. Depression, a debilitating emotional illness, is most frequently described as involving a sense of loss. In the young, the loss is usually due to separation from a parent or the loss of a friend or loved one. In the elderly, however, depression is usually related to a loss of self-esteem, except in those few cases where organic biochemical changes trigger an imbalance in the nervous system (a condition known as endogenous depression or involutional melancholia).

After all, in addition to the loss of loved ones and peers through separation or death, the elderly may encounter other losses almost simultaneously. Not only do they experience a reduction in their physical powers, but also, through retirement, they must face the loss of employment and the feelings of self-worth and status that working provides. All these losses may lead to a depression in which loss of memory, often the major complaint in depressed elderly, is a temporary symptom.

In addition, recent-memory difficulties in the young or old can follow a hospitalization in which the patient received anesthesia or an aggressive course of pain-killing drugs. Upon awakening from anesthesia after an operation, one can experience a tremendous amount of confusion— we actually don't know what has happened when we were unconscious. While in this state of confusion, some loss of memory may occur, but the memory will eventually be recovered.

Gerontologists suggest that loss of recent memory is not necessarily indicative of growing older. Many people of 60 or older find that while they learn and remember more slowly, actual memory loss is uncommon. When our ability to recall slows down, as often happens when we get older, we may perceive that process as increased forgetfulness. In fact, three-quarters of those elderly people who complain about losing their memories are found, upon closer examination, to have normal memories for their age.

Actually, a high percentage of the recent-memory problems experienced by those over the age of 60 are not memory loss but memory lapse, temporary and reversible. The cruel stereotype of senility that makes memory loss appear inevitable and permanent can discourage people from seekingly early diagnosis and proper treatment.

As we have already noted, memory loss can be a symptom of a number of treatable illnesses. Other forms of reversible memory loss may be caused by the very medications that are designed to relieve these symptoms. An older person's brain has been exposed to certain physical changes that make it more vulnerable to the actions and interactions of the body's own chemicals (as, for example, in renal disease, diabetes, or metabolic disorders). The elderly brain is also vulnerable to the chemicals in medications and can be keenly sensitive to drugs even in moderate amounts. There are chemicals in some drugs that react synergistically, multiplying their effects and dulling the brain's response. A frequently cited example of such synergy is the often deadly mixture of tranquilizers and sleeping pills, or the combination of these with alcohol. Drugs that appear to be benign may also induce serious side effects, depending on the body's ability to utilize them.

Memory impairment can also characterize an emotional state in which the patient seems to be suffering from confusion and disorientation. Suppose that an older person whose husband or wife has died is forced to sell the family house but can't go to live with any of the children. With few other choices available, he or she might enter a nursing home. If that institution's staff members are overworked or disinterested (as they might be), they may give the new resident very little help in learning how to adjust to the new environment. Thus the older person must learn where the activity rooms are, at what hour meals are served, what his or her rights as a resident are, how to make a complaint, and the basic rules of the home. It's not difficult to understand how, with such an underwhelming reception, the new resident could become depressed, confused, or disoriented. (In this situation, functional senility can be reversed through psychotherapy.)

In a new living situation that is unfamiliar, symptoms of memory loss are readily apparent. However, when a victim of memory impairment is still in familiar surroundings and continuing to observe the habits of a lifetime, it is sometimes very difficult for other family members to recognize the effects of memory loss. Usually the person who suffers memory loss has some beginning awareness of his impairment, although he may or may not share his concerns with others. When the cause of the memory impairment is organic, as with Alzheimer's disease, early diagnosis can lead to treatment that will help the patient to develop compensatory ways of dealing with his forgetfulness. It also gives the family a better opportunity to deal with the patient's problems and prepare to manage his care successfully.

Determining the cause of some memory impairment is possible through a complete battery of neurological, psychological and physical examinations, preferably at a well-equipped diagnostic center. Alzheimer's, however, can only be confirmed by brain biopsy or an autopsy.

Family members should be alert to early signs of memory loss in their relatives and in themselves. In the earliest stages of a memory-impairing illness, for example, forgetting the names of familiar people and forgetting where objects like keys are placed is the beginning of the process of forgetfulness. This may be ameliorated by setting aside specific places for things, such as a hook near the door for keys. But if the forgetfulness persists and grows worse, it is cause for concern. Some people have difficulty concentrating on a single project: they may find it impossible to pay attention to a television program or a luncheon speaker and become restless and impatient.

Sometimes there are clues in an older person's use of language. At first he may forget words, and later, forget ordinary grammar. Many people seem to have difficulty with numbers—counting, telling time, keeping track of the checkbook balance or the change in their wallets. Other aspects of abstract reasoning, such as the ability to solve problems, also deteriorate.

Perhaps the most obvious symptom, forgetfulness—forgetting where the keys are, doing the same errand twice, sending two or three letters to the same person in a day—is often ignored by physicians and family members because old age is commonly associated with absentmindedness—in short, with "senility."

Usually the victim of memory loss is not aware of it before it is noticed by close family members, friends, or co-workers. The person who *does* fear that he may be developing a permanently disabling illness may deny his forgetfulness by avoiding people or hide it by cuing others to mention their names first, by changing the subject, or by relying on written reminders, which is what Mr. Watson did.

"My husband was a list maker all his life . . . terribly well organized. Whenever we went to the accountant for our taxes, he always had a list of questions all written out. He knew exactly what he wanted to pack when he was going on a trip—always made a list. He's still making lists. I put things down for him, he puts things down for me. The lists are all over the house! But now they don't seem to help. He'll ask me, 'Is this the right list? Is this what I'm looking for?'

"Occasionally I have to go into his desk. There I find shopping lists from weeks before which he's never used, notes to call people which he's never looked at. He doesn't recall that he's recorded these things. It's futile for him to write things down because they serve no purpose. Maybe the lists are defeating a purpose. If he stops thinking about things the moment he writes them down, maybe that's the end of his need to recall."

A common characteristic of all cases of Alzheimer's disease is its effect on recent memory. Recent memory is not the same thing as immediate memory, which refers to the short amount of time it takes to look at a telephone number and then to dial it, for instance. Nor is it *remote memory*, the term given to long-term remembrances from childhood and adolescence. Remote memory is normally permanent and may last a lifetime. Recent memory refers to the events between a few minutes ago and several days in the immediate past.

Not all recent memory is affected. The patient does have memory for certain sensations, such as pain. On the other hand, long-term memories may decay as well. The inconsistent nature of memory loss, both its randomness and its unpredictability, is illustrated by the experience of John Nash.

Mr. Nash is in his early seventies and has had Alzheimer's disease for about three years. Formerly a very conscientious, even dapper dresser, he can no longer remember where his shirts are kept and often wears mismatched socks. He'll belligerently repeat, "Where are my socks?" to his wife over and over again, no matter how many times she shows him. Sometimes, when they are in company with old friends, he will point to an acquaintance of twenty years' standing and ask his wife, "Who is that?"

Yet he was still able to hold a job as a messenger for a mail delivery office. He could get on a bus and go to his office every day. Once at the office, he could then go to another location, collect or deliver a package, and return. However, one day his boss asked him to make a second stop before returning to the office. At that point Mr. Nash announced, "I'm going home." When he got home he told his wife, "I'm not going back there any more."

Mrs. Nash called her husband's office and learned from his employer that he had been fired for refusing to make any second stops. She knew that it would be useless to protest since she had never been able to bring herself to tell the boss, who was in fact an old family friend, about her husband's illness. Now it was too late. She also understood why her husband had refused the extra stops. He was afraid either that he would not be able to find the second address or that he might get lost while looking for and returning from an unfamiliar location. At the same time, Mr. Nash was denying the existence of his problem by refusing to admit to his employer the real reason that he didn't want to make the extra stops.

Getting lost, even in familiar surroundings, is another frequent experience of the person with Alzheimer's disease. Mr. Axelrod was fortunate when he lost his bearings one day.

"Until seven or eight months ago," reported Mrs. Axelrod, who lives in a fashionable section of Washington, "my husband walked out alone, and I let him. Then one day he was gone for about two hours and I became apprehensive. I felt I couldn't leave the house to look for him—what if the police or someone should pick him up and call? But he showed up, and he was still lucid then, too, and he said he got lost and then found.

"We live on a large and busy boulevard, and Mitch found himself somewhere on an isolated street near the river. Because he has a slight limp he walks with a cane and tires easily. Mitch saw a man working on the motor of his car and approached him, told the man that he was tired, and asked if he could sit down inside the car. The man said 'Certainly,' so my husband sat in the car.

"After a few minutes, the man said to him (and my husband remembered and repeated this to me), 'Where do you live?' Mitch couldn't tell him, but luckily he had some identification in his wallet, and the man drove him home. Mitch was a very lucky man. After that I knew he couldn't go out alone, although he didn't know it. I now have a companion who comes in and takes him for walks. They call it an escort service."

While in Mr. Axelrod's case it was already known that he suffered from Alzheimer's disease, many families deny the illness of the spouse or parent until a dramatic event occurs, such as getting lost. Many Alzheimer's patients don't know their address and become very upset when they get lost.

Travel outside the home presents other dangers as well. Most caregivers soon recognize that they must take over the car and all the driving. Yet even that solution does not eliminate all problems. Carla Esses recalls:

"I was driving us to my daughter's one Sunday. We were on the highway, doing about 60 miles an hour, when my husband, in the passenger seat, decided to get out of the car and suddenly opened the door! He had forgotten that the car was moving."

Mrs. Esses has changed the lock so that the passenger door may be opened only from the outside and now goes around to the passenger side to let her husband in and out.

Dangers to the patient in the outside world are matched by dangers at home. Stories of patients who have turned on a gas jet or stove burner and then forgotten it are all too frequent. Many families restrict the patient's access to the kitchen stove and to dangerous power tools.

Confusion, or "getting lost," happens at home, too. Posting a photograph of a bathroom on the bathroom door helps the Alzheimer's patient find his way around the house. Caregivers put labels in oversize letters, such as HENRY'S ROOM, on the door to the person's room. And they label everything: locations of clothes in drawers and closets, silverware in a kitchen drawer, shelves where plates are kept. While it requires considerable effort to take these measures, there are rewards for both the patient and the caregivers. The Alzheimer's patient is helped and reassured by such a highly structured environment. Using visual aids, the patient can do simple household tasks such as drying the dishes or, in the early stage, putting things away. Not only does such activity help to bolster the patient's self-esteem, it also relieves, at least for a while, the pressure on the caregivers to do absolutely every housekeeping chore.

Although the patient may not say what pleases, concerns, or reassures him, family members must assume that he is aware of his forgetfulness and is relieved when labels and frequent visual clues reduce the number of things to remember.

Even people who consider their memories to be perfectly reliable resort to memory aids such as lists, notes on bulletin boards, wrist alarms, and other reminders. Expanding those techniques to assist someone in the house who is memory-impaired is one of the ways in which a family caregiver can be helpful and contribute to the patient's sense of well-being. Managing problem behaviors will be fully discussed in the second part of this book.

It is also very helpful for caregivers to learn as much as they can about the nature of the disease, the way it is diagnosed, and what researchers have been able to discover about the specific characteristics of Alzheimer's disease.

CHAPTER 2

Alzheimer's Disease: What It Is and What It Is Not

*A*lzheimer's disease, which accounts for more than half of all the victims of organically caused memory loss, is named for the German physician Alois Alzheimer, who first described the disease in the early 1900s. He identified a presenile form of the illness occurring in people as young as age 30. Later research found that a milder but more common form of the disease affected older people. Today, Alzheimer's disease is labeled *senile dementia—Alzheimer's type,* generally abbreviated SDAT.

Alzheimer's disease is the fourth most prevalent cause of death—after heart disease, cancer, and stroke. Death certificates now denote Alzheimer's disease as the cause of death; as with cancer, it is failure of an organ (the brain in this case) that causes death. In the past deaths from Alzheimer's disease were usually ascribed to pneumonia. The life expectancy of an Alzheimer's patient is reduced by up to one-third when matched for age to other elderly people.

The loss of intellectual abilities is of sufficient severity to interfere with everyday social and occupational functioning. The victim's capacity to think abstractly is impaired; he is unable to find similarities and differences between related words and has trouble defining words and concepts. His judgment is also impaired. There may be disturbances in language (aphasia), an inability to carry out motor activities (apraxia), or a failure to recognize or identify objects despite intact sensory and motor functions of the brain (agnosia). An alteration of personality or accentuation of traits that existed prior to the onset of the illness (premorbid traits) also occurs eventually. The onset of Alzheimer's disease (known technically as *primary degenerative dementia*) is insidious with uniformly progressive deterioration. Presenile onset is between the ages of 40 and 60, senile onset is after age 65.

A study conducted in the 1980s by Denyse Gautrin, et al. regarding the prevalence of Alzheimer's disease in the general population indicated the rates were:

ages 65–74	1%
ages 75–84	4%
ages 85+	10.5%

or approximately 75,000 new cases worldwide in 1986. Projections for the year 2016 are estimated to be over 215,000.[1]

Changes within the Brain

Medical evidence presumes or indicates there is a specific organic factor judged to be etiologically related to the disturbance. Alzheimer identified and described a patient in middle age whose behavior gradually deteriorated into jealousy. Later on, other behavioral changes, such as paranoia and intellectual and memory disturbances, were seen in people whose illness was in the advanced stages. The forehead (frontal lobes) and inside of the temples (temporal lobes) have the most severe brain decompensation; this can only be seen upon autopsy.

Since Alzheimer's early discoveries, scientists have studied the pathology that occurs in the inner and outer layers of the brain and is also found in brain tissue and nerve cells. There are three characteristics that

1. Denyse Gautrin, Sorona Frode, Hugues Tetreault, et al. (University of Quebec INRS, Sante, Montreal), "Canadian Projection of Cases Suffering from Alzheimer's Disease and Senile Dementia of Alzheimer's Type over Period 1986–2031," *Canadian Journal of Psychology* 35, no. 2 (March 1990): 166.

suggest brain changes. First and most important are neurofibrillary tangles (an accumulation of abnormal fibers concentrated in the cytoplasm of a cell). Under the electron microscope, these fibers appear as a tangle of filaments. The tangles occur most densely in an area of the brain known as the hippocampus. Recent or short-term memory is associated with this area, which is also part of a system called the limbic system (otherwise known as the "seat of the emotions").

The outer cortex, known as the parietal association cortex, is the next area affected. This part of the brain helps a person to understand information taken in by the five senses. Also associated with damage to this area is the loss of language ability and the inability to remember things like how to find the toilet in your own home or how to put on your clothing. Lastly, the area of the brain controlling the total personality is affected when the frontal association cortex withers and dies.

A change that can also be seen in brain tissue under the electron microscope consists of neuritic plaques or aggregations of degenerated neural material. Granulovascular degeneration is the third pathological change that occurs in the interior of a cell; the cell becomes filled with vacuoles that have fluid and granular material.[2] As there is increased granulovascular degeneration, there appears to be increased loss of mental function.

A protein, beta-amyloid, has been implicated as the cause of senile plaques in the brain. This protein has also been found in the skin and intestines of Alzheimer's victims. Beta-amyloid protein triggers tissue damage by causing nerve cells to sprout abnormally. They look like loose bundles of long, thin fibers when placed under the electron microscope. Although beta-amyloid protein is secreted naturally in many parts of the brain and other parts of the body, it causes damage primarily in the cerebral cortex.

Modern scientists have also identified some of the chemical changes that occur in the brains of those affected with Alzheimer's disease. In order to function, different parts of the brain cells and neurons must

2. Reprinted with permission of The Free Press, a division of Macmillan Publishing Company, from *Brain Failure* by Barry Reisberg. Copyright © 1981 by Barry Reisberg, M.D.

communicate with each other. The communication depends on electrical impulses that are the product of neurochemical interactions. The chemical that leads to communication between the nerve cells is known as a neurotransmitter.

One important neurotransmitter, acetylcholine (ACH), is produced by the enzyme choline acetyltransferase (CAT). If CAT levels in the brain drop by as much as 90 percent, the level of ACH in the hippocampus and the cerebral cortex is badly reduced; the brain does not have enough ACH for memory formation. Researchers are trying to develop therapies to restore a safe level of acetylcholine. The danger is that excessive amounts of this chemical in the brain induce nightmares, confusion, agitation, and slower intellectual and motor functions; at even higher accumulations, ACH can produce decreased blood pressure, reduced heart rate, and paralysis of the muscles necessary for breathing, resulting in death.

When groups of nerve endings scattered throughout the cortex degenerate, the resulting areas of degenerated neural material disrupt the passage of electrochemical signals between the cells. Under the microscope, these areas appear to be plaques. The greater the number of neuritic plaques and neurofibrillary tangles, the more disturbed is intellectual functioning and memory.

The mutation of the gene involved with the production of the normal brain protein, beta-amyloid, can also cause Alzheimer's disease. Fragments of this protein are found accumulating in sticky balls outside the dying or dead cells in the brain. This suggests that fragments of beta-amyloid can kill brain cells that control memory and reasoning. It is only *after* the beta-amyloid fragments attach themselves to brain cells that the cells die. The therapy of the future may ultimately be to block beta-amyloid with enzymes. Now we are faced with more definitive evidence that Alzheimer's is truly a disease characterized by a specific pattern of nerve cell death.

Besides the chemical changes, the brain's size and shape alters. The constant loss of brain cells is so accelerated in the person with Alzheimer's disease that the brain shrinks and appears to be a very aged brain. At the same time, the ventricles (inner spaces) of the brain increase in size and the outer layer of cells becomes less dense and thinner.

Characteristics of the Disease

Researchers report data that support a common genetic factor for familial Alzheimer's disease. The possibility that a relationship exists between the mother's age at pregnancy and the disease has been speculated; however, not enough research exists to verify this. There is a slightly greater incidence of Alzheimer's disease in families that have been affected by the disorder.

It is an intrinsic characteristic of Alzheimer's disease that the symptoms vary from patient to patient, and sometimes from day to day in the same patient. In discussing Alzheimer's disease, we saturate each statement with qualifying words such as *often, tends, perhaps, some, probably,* and *may,* emphasizing our realization that no single symptom or behavior is completely predictable. However, the loss of recent memory seems to be a universal symptom.

This capricious variability is among the most frustrating aspects of day-to-day life with an Alzheimer's patient. After days of garbling words and speaking sentences that sound nonsensical, the patient may suddenly have a lucid interval and carry on a conversation that appears in every way to be normal. The respite is usually temporary, and soon the gibberish returns. Now, however, the patient's family is left even more uncertain, confused, and chagrined. Is there hope? How can we treat Aunt Susan like a dysfunctional person when we can see glimpses of her mind still operating within? What makes her aware one moment and disoriented and helpless at other times? Loss of memory is such a painful source of distress because without memory we don't know if we have loved or felt pleasure, sorrow, or regret. We also don't know if we are loved, and our sense of security and reliability is so shaken that we become anxious and afraid even of those people on whom we once could depend.

Symptoms that all normal people experience from time to time are also experienced by the patient with Alzheimer's disease. Generally, fever, fatigue, or achiness is the result of physical illness or some feeling of emotional malaise due to frustration or depression. Most of us recover quickly from these symptoms. But the person with Alzheimer's disease does not recover quickly; indeed, as the illness progresses, there is a steady mental and physical deterioration that usually occurs slowly over time (sometimes several years), although in some cases the progression occurs rapidly.

Possible Causes of Alzheimer's Disease

Research over the past thirty years has uncovered a great deal of information about Alzheimer's disease, but researchers do not yet know exactly why certain people develop the disease and many others do not. They have ruled out a link to intellectual capacity, social or economic class, or occupation.

In recent years it has become increasingly clear that genetic factors play a part in the development of Alzheimer's disease; around one-third of all cases seem to be inherited through a dominant gene. Researchers agree that about 10 to 15 percent of the general population has a genetic predisposition to developing Alzheimer's disease. In 1991 one scientific journal reported that this percentage could be higher. There is also a theory, still controversial, that differing patterns of Alzheimer's disease mean that some families are more likely to develop it than others. For some families the risk that siblings or children will develop the disease after age 85 could be as high as 50 percent, whereas for others the risk is zero.

Although some families may have more than one member with Alzheimer's disease, it is difficult to determine whether the disease will be inherited by others, especially if its onset occurs very late in life. It is believed that most close family members of an Alzheimer's patient won't develop the disease, but they run a risk that is twice that of the general population. Information gathered on 200 siblings of Alzheimer's patients indicates that identical twin siblings (who have identical genes) are expected to develop the disease. Fraternal twins (who share many of the same genes, but not all) have a 50 percent chance. However, genetic factors only create a predisposition to developing the disease; they don't necessarily cause it.

In 1987 scientists isolated one gene that is involved in Alzheimer's disease on chromosome 21. In 1990 a gene on chromosome 19 was also implicated, and it is now believed that a third gene can cause the disease. Attention has focused on the gene involved in producing the brain protein beta-amyloid. The mutation of this gene can cause overproduction of beta-amyloid, which may damage the brain cells that control memory and reasoning.

Clinical evidence suggests that catastrophic life circumstances can lead to unremitting stress. Although there are no conclusive hard data to verify this hypothesis, the possibility has been raised that stress may play a role in the onset of Alzheimer's disease. The death of a loved one followed by a sequence of mourning is one of the most stressful human experiences. Failure to work through and achieve recovery from the loss of a loved one during the final stages of the mourning process is an indication of the continued state of stress that the individual is under. People who have not recovered from such an experience within a reasonable period of time (approximately one year) seem to be more vulnerable to a catastrophic illness more frequently. Continued stress eventually affects the endocrine, immune, and nervous systems. Visible signs of the illness are first reflected in the biological "Achilles heel" or most vulnerable area of the person. Aging behavior becomes accelerated, resistance to viral and bacterial infection decreases, allergic reactions are accentuated, and the immune system is not as effective. The incidence of cancer increases. Emotional breakdown and mental collapse may also be the accompanying psychological components of persisting unrelieved stress.[3]

And what about that familiar term, "hardening of the arteries"? Is there such a thing, and what is it? The term is almost synonymous with

3. Reprinted from Thomas Crook and Samuel Gershon, eds., *Strategies for the Development of an Effective Treatment for Senile Dementia* (New Canaan, CT: Mark Powley Assoc., Inc., 1981).

19

senility and has many of the same connotations. However, recent medical discoveries now show that very few—no more than 10 percent—of the cases of organically related memory loss are caused either by arteriosclerosis (hardening of the blood vessel walls) or by atherosclerosis (narrowing, closing, or thickening of the interior blood vessel walls due to fatty deposits). Fatty deposits are almost always present to some degree in the circulatory systems of middle-aged and elderly people. Damage to the brain may occur when the blood flow is so restricted that insufficient oxygen and nutrients are carried to the brain.

Various types of stroke-related pathology—including diffusely distributed micro-infarcts—are more apt to be implicated in senile dementia.

Describing the mental deterioration of an older person as due to "cerebral atherosclerosis" is thus a medical misdiagnosis.

Cholesterol does not seem to play a part in Alzheimer's disease. In fact, the cholesterol content of a brain affected by Alzheimer's is typically lower than that of an unaffected brain of similar age. Cholesterol is important in the normal growth and functioning of brain nerve cells. Brain cells can make cholesterol even if they don't get enough from the serum cholesterol in the blood, but the relationship between these types of cholesterol has not been fully studied.

Phases of Alzheimer's Disease

Although each individual is different, there are several identifiable phases of the illness, each with its own set of symptoms.

The onset of Alzheimer's disease is insidious, meaning that its effects appear gradually. At first there is no decrease in function and no sign of cognitive decline. Then a person starts to complain of forgetting where he puts things.

"Where are those darn keys?" asks Miss Lucy Baines. "And my purse and eyeglasses? They were just here in my hands." She looks mournfully around and turns her room upside down but still doesn't find them.

Relatives may not be sure that anything is wrong with the person. He may seem to have less energy, drive, and initiative and be slower to react and to learn new things. In the beginning stages of Alzheimer's the patient seeks and prefers familiar people, places, and things, like Mr. Saints:

> MRS. ALMA SAINTS: "These days, all we do on Sunday is go visiting—mostly we visit the family. We don't go to see friends, although they invite us, because Max usually begs off. He doesn't enjoy any of the things we used to do. The only people we really see regularly are my brother and his wife. They are quiet people and Max has always liked them."

Mr. Saints avoids unfamiliar situations that may be too much for him to handle and seems to be less discriminating than before. Miss Baines faces a greater challenge, experiencing difficulty maintaining her daily routine. Even more disruptive is a catastrophic reaction to forgetting things, becoming anxious and angry. Clarence Havermeyer describes such a story about his father:

> "Dad used to be a champ at word games. He was a great reader and he loved crossword puzzles and the English language. One day we were talking about witchcraft, and he kept looking for a word to describe Satan. I came up with words like 'devil, wicked.' He said 'Mephistopheles,' but there was another word like devilish and he just couldn't think of it. He kept saying 'dev-den.' I couldn't think of it either. But Dad got so irritated that he stormed out of the room to the kitchen and barked at my mother, 'Let's go home!' I never saw him so upset! Just over a word! I guess he meant 'demonic'; I looked it up in *Roget's Thesaurus* and called to tell him, but he wouldn't come to the phone. Poor Dad!"

The next phase of the illness brings with it decreased ability to perform complex tasks, such as planning a dinner party, marketing, or handling finances. The Alzheimer's patient may misunderstand what he hears, lose the thread of a story, or miss the punch line of a simple joke. He may be unable to calculate and may need help with the checkbook. There is mild to moderate intellectual decline. Mrs. Frost had a tough time when her husband entered this stage:

"You don't know what I went through with the damned checkbook! He would give me money for food. Sometimes I spent thirty dollars a week, then maybe I'd need forty or fifty dollars a week for food, what with inflation. When I asked for more, he'd get angry. It wasn't that he didn't have any more to give me. It was simply that he was afraid to write checks. So instead he would give me a big argument and tell me that I was reckless with money. For six months he hid the fact that he couldn't balance the checkbook anymore before he finally gave it up and asked me to take over. By that time, he was very confused."

In this stage of the illness there are more losses. Planning ahead and making decisions become very troublesome tasks, as they did for Mr. Skolnick. His daughter told us that the illness came on so gradually that she wasn't aware of it. They were partners in their grocery business, and she depended on him all the time. Suddenly, he couldn't make decisions about how many cases of tuna or toilet paper to order. In the beginning, her father denied that there was any problem. When she finally realized something was wrong, she felt helpless and didn't know what to do.

Increasingly self-absorbed, the impaired person seems totally insensitive to the needs and feelings of other people; he seems to avoid any situations that may end in failure. The person in this phase is continuing to function but may need some supervision.

Obvious disability marks the middle stage of dementia. The victim of Alzheimer's disease loses his orientation to time and place, and he is not able to identify familiar people or events. It happened to Mr. Kenyon:

"My husband and I went to our grandson's birthday party. He didn't want to go, but I said, 'We're going,' and I didn't give him an alternative. At the party he had fun; he laughed and joked. He has a terrific sense of humor, and he remembers things that happened years and years ago. He had a good time. On the way home he admitted that. The next day I mentioned some of the nice people who were at the party. He said, 'What party?' I was stunned. I couldn't believe it. He had totally forgotten about the party as if he'd never been there."

As described by his wife, Mr. Kenyon is now obviously disabled. He is very lethargic, invents words of his own, and needs repeated instruction and direction. He cannot choose proper clothing by himself and must be coaxed to bathe. He needs help to go to the toilet. Unsure of himself, he behaves in unexpected ways and expresses very little warmth to people with whom he has had close relationships. While his memory of recent events fails, he seems to recall the past with astonishing clarity. There is considerable change in his behavior, some of which is exaggerated and often bizarre.

In a further phase of the illness the victim is apathetic and unable to find his way around a familiar house or apartment. He wanders and needs help with all of the activities that encompass daily life and self-care.

Mr. Cook tells about his ordeal.

"My wife and I used to enjoy eating dinner out at least three times a week. Now, because there are problems with eating, we don't go out to dinner anymore. I can't take her out because I have to spoon-feed her. What fun is that? I also have to hold her hands because the hands are all over. They are either messing in the food, or knocking over a glass, or spilling the coffee. I'm too uncomfortable and embarrassed to go out to dinner with her anymore."

The impaired person continues to lose recent and remote memories. There is very severe cognitive decline. Syllables, words, and phrases are repeated over and over. He does not recognize himself in the mirror, nor does he recognize other people. That happened to Mr. Florio.

"My husband used to play cards with a group of other fellows one day a week. Now, he'll meet one of them who will ask 'How are you? How're you feeling?' or whatever. Then he'll walk away, and I'll say to my husband, 'Don't you remember him? You played cards every week.' He doesn't remember anybody."

Also in this phase of Alzheimer's disease, depression, delusions, or delirium may occur. With the gradual memory loss comes loss of personal dignity followed by lack of confidence. The impaired person may become incontinent, lose all intelligible speech, and become stuporous or comatose.

A rating scale used to diagnose progressive impairments in a patient's functioning has shown that the first impaired function is often the ability to manage finances. This is followed by an inability to select clothing, dress, or bathe without assistance. In the last stages, speech and motor abilities are lost progressively; speech may become limited to half a dozen words and then diminish to one word that becomes the response to all questions. The ability to move about and sit up decreases, and there are gait problems. The final function that is lost is the ability to smile.

Just as it takes a child a few months or longer to learn a skill, so the Alzheimer's victim tends to lose skills within a similar time frame. The abilities to walk, talk, and do personal tasks are lost in the reverse order in which they were learned in childhood. For example, an eleven-month-old child who cannot yet walk is often not yet able to speak in sentences. Similarly, when an Alzheimer's patient can no longer walk, he loses the ability to speak in sentences. Each layer of developmental skills acquired from childhood onward is slowly peeled away.

Diseases with Similar Symptoms

Many of the same stages and symptoms that characterize Alzheimer's disease are also noticeable in patients with multi-infarct dementia (MID). Because the destruction of neural material takes place in a somewhat different way, MID can be differentiated from Alzheimer's disease through autopsy. In an autopsy, the brains of MID victims show areas of cerebral softening, also known as stroke areas. Researchers believe that these areas are produced by multiple infarctions. An infarction is a patch of dead or damaged tissue and is the result of a ministroke, or many little strokes. These tiny strokes happen when atherosclerotic matter travels to the brain from other parts of the body and blocks the flow of blood to the brain.

By itself, multi-infarct dementia afflicts 15 percent of all victims of organic brain syndrome. Combined, multi-infarct dementia and Alzheimer's disease account for as much as 90 percent of all organic brain disorders.

Despite their common symptom, loss of recent memory, there are notable differences between multi-infarct dementia and Alzheimer's disease. Most important is the evident cardiovascular connection in multi-infarct dementia. The same predisposing factors associated with cardiovascular arteriosclerosis also seem to be operating in multi-infarct dementia. Heart attack, angina pectoris, hypertension, diabetes mellitus, obesity, vascular disease, and cigarette smoking have all been implicated in MID.

As opposed to the gradual appearance of Alzheimer's disease, the onset of multi-infarct dementia is likely to be sudden and abrupt. There are certain periods of rapid worsening and some improvement from strokes. People who have had strokes may recover after rehabilitative training. Alzheimer's sufferers, on the other hand, seem to decline gradually, experiencing only subtle changes but no improvement over many years. They also, unlike most MID victims, show fluctuations in behavior that may be both diverse and unpredictable.

Although men and women may be equally affected by MID and Alzheimer's disease, more women seem to be afflicted by Alzheimer's disease simply because women outlive men by seven to twelve years. Multi-infarct dementia generally appears earlier, between the ages of 40 and 60, while the age of onset of Alzheimer's disease is usually over 65.

Other conditions that have as their major symptoms confused behavior and loss of recent memory, but that afflict far fewer people, include Huntington's disease, certain types of Parkinson's disease, Creutzfield-Jacob's disease, and Pick's disease. Of these, the symptoms of Pick's disease most closely resemble those of Alzheimer's disease, making the two extremely difficult to differentiate except by autopsy. The characteristic changes in nerve cells are concentrated in the frontal lobe of the brain in Pick's disease, and the average age of onset is much younger— as early as 40 or 50. A victim of Pick's disease lacks initiative and will become continually more passive until he becomes a "vegetable" with no remaining memory. Alzheimer's victims, however, generally retain some memory and are at times agitated and hyperactive.

The following problems may also cause or mimic signs of dementia: depression, head injuries, nutritional deficiencies, brain tumors, adverse drug reactions, thyroid problems, and hydrocephalies. Infections such as meningitis, syphilis, or auto-immune deficiency syndrome (AIDS) may also be suspect. In fact, dementia may be caused by any infection involving the brain.

CHAPTER 3

Diagnosing Alzheimer's Disease

*U*ntil recently, the general term used to describe memory-impaired behavior when there is no discernible physical cause was *organic brain syndrome*. The new terminology used to describe patients over the age of 65 who are confused and disoriented and show intellectual and memory impairment, bizarre behavior, and shallow emotional reactions is senile dementia. Neurobiological experts suggest that senile dementia can be a temporary state that can be treated and reversed or a permanent (irreversible) condition that results from physical changes in the brain.

Factors in the Disease

Familial factors and Down's syndrome (Mongolism) as well as age itself are implicated in the development of Alzheimer's disease. Aging itself can cause damage to the chromosomes, damage that may also be caused by hazards in the environment or by a slow viral infection that spreads from one member of a family to another.

There is a strong association between Down's syndrome, a genetic disease caused by an extra chromosome, and Alzheimer's disease. A statistically significant study indicates that there are similar fingerprint patterns in people with Alzheimer's and Down's syndrome. Furthermore, nearly all those born with Down's syndrome who live past the age of 35 go on to develop Alzheimer's disease. Although this link needs further scientific investigation and confirmation, there seems to be a genetic vulnerability factor for Alzheimer's patients and their families.[4]

Many different conditions, including nutritional deficiencies, chemical imbalances in the blood, tumors, and environmental stressors such as metal poisoning from manganese or aluminum, may also lead to the symptoms of recent-memory loss. In particular, aluminum salts are found in everything we eat, including food, vitamins, and antacids. Although dying neurons seem to collect aluminum, we do not know whether the accumulation is a cause or an effect of Alzheimer's disease.

A few of the more common causes of memory impairment were discussed in the previous chapter. Because so many of these potential conditions are treatable if discovered in time, neurological, psychological, and medical evaluations are necessary to rule them out as the major cause of the memory loss, disoriented and confused behavior, impaired judgment, and shallow emotional reactions typical of the Alzheimer's patient. The purpose of the diagnostic tests is to find a cause other than degenerative progressive damage to the brain. Therefore, the diagnosis of Alzheimer's disease is one of excluding other conditions that may produce similar symptoms, including memory loss. For example, it is important to differentiate depression from Alzheimer's disease.

A differential diagnosis helps to clarify whether depression is causing the patient to look and act as if he were demented or whether the patient experiencing a dementing illness is also depressed. Depressed people express feelings of anxiety; they underestimate their real abilities, have low self-esteem, and move and speak slowly. They appear to have memory gaps and poor intellectual functioning. However, when they receive treatment for depression, memory improves and intellectual functioning also improves. By contrast, the Alzheimer's patient usually denies his decrease in intellectual areas and memory. The depressed person tends to exaggerate his sense of distress, whereas the Alzheimer's patient

---

4. Personal communication from Richard Moles, Ph.D., Associate Professor of Psychiatry, Mount Sinai School of Medicine, New York, NY.

shows little emotional reaction. When depression and Alzheimer's disease exist simultaneously, the person may be successfully treated with antidepressants. He will become less depressed; however, his memory and intellectual functioning will *not* be restored despite the treatment.

Identifying the sleep patterns of Alzheimer's patients can also be useful in helping clinicians distinguish Alzheimer's disease from depression. Alzheimer's patients tend to take a much longer time to reach REM sleep (the sleep stage of rapid eye movement when dreaming occurs) than do normal aging subjects. Depressed people, however, reach REM sleep in less time than do normal aging subjects. Other sleep patterns characteristic of Alzheimer's disease include sundown syndrome, a pattern of delirious behavior in which the patient wakes up while others are sleeping and is confused, agitated, and active; and sleep apnea, a disorder in which breathing virtually stops (accompanied by a decrease of oxygen saturation of the blood) during portions of sleep. In general, Alzheimer's patients awaken more often and do not sleep as deeply as healthy older people.

A critical issue in the diagnosis of depression is a family or personal history of depression, previous episodes of depression, or a history of manic-depressive illness. Endogenous depression (involutional melancholia due to biochemical changes in the nervous system) comes about acutely; Alzheimer's disease has an insidious onset. The depressed person's memory loss may be the result of loneliness after the loss of a spouse or a disappointment in himself, another, or his fate. Rewarding human contact and beneficial activity will help to restore his sense of well-being. The Alzheimer's patient may be tenderly cared for and still become anxious, fearful, and enraged at caregivers.

Diagnostic Tests

Gerontological researchers, working together with neurologists, psychologists, and psychotherapists, have in recent years developed a basic diagnostic approach to evaluating the person with suspected Alzheimer's disease. Traditional techniques are combined with sophisticated

29

technological instruments to evaluate the person suspected of having a memory-impairing disease.

A family physician in general practice, an internist, a neurologist, or a psychiatrist may order these diagnostic tests or suggest consultation with a professional who will both supervise and interpret the test results to the family. Most important is that there be one professional person who will take responsibility for ordering the tests and then evaluating the results of all of the diagnostic procedures. As a member of the patient's family, it is important that you feel comfortable with that person and free enough to ask the most delicate and intimate questions to which you can anticipate receiving clear and thoughtful answers. Due to the prohibitive cost of some diagnostic equipment, part if not all of the comprehensive evaluation must be performed at a major medical center specializing in disorders of the brain.

A typical basic evaluation of a patient with suspected Alzheimer's disease usually includes the following:[5]

A social and medical history taken from the patient and from a relative or friend will disclose any prior conditions such as loss of a loved one, toxic exposure, or infection that could be implicated in the patient's current confusion.

A thorough physical examination will be conducted, including a *neuro-psychological examination* that tests sensory and motor functions, the mental status of the patient, and his psychological capacities including verbal, intellectual, and reasoning abilities.

In the sensory portion of the examination, a neurologist may, for example, test the patient's sensitivity to pain with a pinprick. Other sensory tests determine hearing impairment, a frequent cause of confusion in older people.

Motor ability, such as balance and the symmetry and briskness of reflexes, are also tested. Since motor functions are controlled by the frontal lobe of the brain, an unusual response here may suggest a different cause for the memory impairment.

5. Michael A. Jenike, M.D.

The face-hand test is a simple screening procedure that can be used by physicians or psychologists. Sitting face to face with the patient, the examiner asks the patient to close his eyes and then tell where he feels a touch. (Examiner will alternately touch the hands and cheeks of the patient; the same test is done with the eyes opened.) Errors on this test strongly suggest that there is brain damage.

A mental status questionnaire indicates how well the patient is oriented in terms of time, place, and person. It includes ten questions such as "Who is the President of the United States?," "What is today's date?," "What is the year?," and "When is your birthday?" Mental alertness is indicated by a score of ten.

Memory for digits is a test that has been abstracted from an intelligence test and determines the patient's ability to remember and repeat digits forward and then backward. The digits are in a series of from two to eight numbers.

A "misplaced objects" test is usually administered by a psychologist and used less frequently than other tests. The patient is asked to place pictures of familiar objects within representations of typical rooms such as a bedroom, bathroom, or kitchen. This test determines the patient's ability to remember where familiar objects in a room belong, such as a bathtub in a bathroom.

Paper and pencil tests are used by psychologists to evaluate the mental condition of a patient, and a *clinical interview* by a psychologist or a psychiatrist will assist in evaluating the emotional well-being of a patient and screen for emotional illness, including paranoia and depression. Based on the results of the physical and psychological evaluations and the patient's history, doctors may then recommend laboratory tests. These tests should be based on a patient's individual condition, so they will differ from person to person.

CAT (computerized axial tomogram) scan is essentially an X-ray of the structure of the brain. The scanner uses X-rays to construct by computer a picture of the subject's brain. Pathological changes occur in the brain of a person with Alzheimer's disease: brain cells decay faster than those of a normal brain, making the brain appear to be shrunken and to

31

have a thinner outer layer. The decayed neural material concentrates in unusual shapes (the neuritic plaques and neurofibrillary tangles that Alzheimer first identified), and the inner spaces of the brain increase in size. The CAT scan shows the location of decay, the shrinkage of tissue, and the enlarged inner spaces (ventricles). The larger the ventricles, the greater the degree of impairment in memory and day-to-day functioning. While a CAT scan (or two scans made at an interval of a year or more) can indicate neural decay, it can not, by itself, provide an absolute diagnosis of Alzheimer's disease.

Magnetic resonance imaging (MRI) is the latest and most sensitive procedure to detect atrophy of the brain stem, mass lesions, or small infarcts. MRI can also clarify ambiguous CAT scan findings.

The PETT (positron emission transaxial tomography) scan has been used by researchers to study the changes in the brain through a picture of how the brain functions. The scanner monitors the use of a radioisotopic form of glucose by the subject's brain and indicates how varying parts of the brain use the glucose for metabolism and energy. A brain affected by Alzheimer's disease uses less glucose than a normal brain.

EEG (electroencephalogram) measures the electrical activity (brain waves) of the brain. Abnormally slow activity of the brain waves suggests abnormality in the brain mass. Spike activity that is abnormal can suggest epileptic seizures. *A quantitative EEG (QEEG)* is a more valuable test than the conventional EEG because it uses a computer to analyze brain waves. In the Alzheimer's patient the EEG wave bands are slowed (general thinking processes of the Alzheimer's patient are also slowed down). QEEG is used selectively and is not a routine procedure.

Lumbar puncture (spinal tap). In this procedure a small amount of spinal fluid is drawn by a needle inserted between the pelvis and the ribs. Analysis of this fluid, which also surrounds the brain, can detect malignancies, neurosyphilis, and certain kinds of infections that can cause memory loss and are not discoverable by other means. The procedure is frightening to contemplate and difficult to explain to a confused person. Although when performed with local anesthesia it is generally not painful, there may be some uncomfortable aftereffects. Like the EEG, a lumbar puncture is not a standard procedure and should only be used selectively.

Among the many causes of memory impairment that are detectable by a *blood analysis* are thyroid, kidney, and liver malfunctions; certain nutritional deficiencies leading to conditions such as pernicious anemia and pellagra; infections such as tuberculosis; and a variety of metabolic and chemical imbalances. Particular tests may be suggested from clues in the patient's history and physical examination. Others, such as a screening for tuberculosis, are usual procedures but not always necessary.

Some of the tests we have discussed are primarily research tools; however, they are enormously valuable in assessing the degree of impairment and confirming a diagnosis of Alzheimer's disease. Other tests are standard and give information that is also valuable in diagnosis. Certain tests may have to be repeated. Being tested too often may inconvenience and discomfort the Alzheimer's patient, but it is important not to miss signs of the disease.

In very special cases, a brain biopsy may be suggested to look directly into the opened brain rather than through indirect testing. This is a surgical procedure, done under general anesthesia by a neurosurgeon. A small portion of the skull is removed and a sample of brain tissue is taken. The brain biopsy can detect herpes in the brain, a treatable infection that, if ignored, leads to memory impairment and ultimately, in nine out of ten cases, to death. The diagnosis of Alzheimer's disease can also be verified through a brain biopsy; however, since there is no present treatment or cure for the disease, family members and the physician may decide that it is both inappropriate and dangerous to subject the patient to the stress of anesthesia and surgery.

Family members, in their desire to find a way to improve the patient's condition, may insist that every possible test be made at every successive level. In general, additional tests, after the results of the first evaluation are known, are worthwhile only if suggested by the initial screening. Without a specific reason to probe further, the patient is subjected to needless additional risk and suffering and the family must bear unnecessarily increased expenses.

The physician, psychologist, or other specialist who is familiar with your relative's case will assemble the results of all of these tests to explain them to you and other family members. If the reversible physical and psychological reasons for the patient's confusion and forgetfulness have been considered and rejected, the family must face the possibility that a relative has one of several diseases that are collectively referred to as progressive dementing illness. A clearer picture of the nature of the disease and its effects on the patient will enable you to evaluate the alternatives in patient care and management that are available. Still, unless a brain biopsy has been performed, a confirmed diagnosis of Alzheimer's or similar disease can only be made through an autopsy of the patient's brain after his death.

All of the illnesses that cause organic changes in the brain are chronic (except tumors and some infections) and virtually irreversible. Whatever specific name is given to the illness, the personal meaning of the term is clear. Someone who is close to you and whom you love is losing the ability to think and to remember.

CHAPTER 4

Treating the "Silent Epidemic": Research Developments

*I*n recent years, psychologists, psychiatrists, geriatric specialists, neurologists, gerontologists, and nurses have learned more about the progression of Alzheimer's disease. Increased knowledge of the illness has helped them to develop some ideas that can be adapted by caregivers to help the patient live more fully in the early stages of the disability. We cannot yet prevent or cure the disease, nor can we reverse its course; but we can reduce the degree of impairment and improve the quality of the lives of Alzheimer's victims by detecting and treating delusions and depression with medication and behavioral and talk therapies.

Today there is a stronger therapeutic understanding of the patient's suffering and the corresponding burden placed on caregivers. A clearer picture of the family situation enables family members who are caregivers to survive this encounter—an encounter that some families have described as a war. At present, the treatment approach to the person afflicted with Alzheimer's is to help him maintain the maximum amount of dignity and comfort possible. Yet, as more people become vulnerable to Alzheimer's and similar diseases, the search for more active treatment and eventual cure intensifies.

Epidemiologists, who investigate the causes and control of widespread medical epidemics, predict that by the year 2030, when about 20 percent of the population (about 51 million people) will be over the age of 65, the United States will have a "silent epidemic" of Alzheimer's disease.[6] Because of the increased aging, or "graying," of the population of this country, 10 to 20 percent of people over age 65 have clinically significant intellectual impairment.

Dihydroergotoxine mesylate (Hydergine) is a drug prescribed for mild dementia. It was approved by the Federal Food and Drug Administration (FDA) in the mid-1960s and is marketed throughout the United States; however, it is now being reexamined by the FDA. Dihydroergotoxine mesylate is purported to make people feel better and behave better, and although the research was statistically significant, there is no real evidence that it helps basic memory loss symptoms. Although it does not restore brain cells, some specialists on the condition suggest that about 20 percent of the patients taking the drug show improvement in mood, and since there is as yet no alternative, they advocate its use.

In the United States treatment approaches to Alzheimer's and related diseases have lagged behind Europe owing to the conservatism and caution of the FDA. In Western Europe the population may already be older than that of the United States. There, many more drugs are on the market that claim to treat Alzheimer's disease, regardless of whether or not they are effective. Some drugs have been used as treatment for mental functioning, including cerebral vasodilators that increase blood circulation to the brain, but this does not help the memory and seems ineffective. Gerovital H-3, obtained from Rumania and now available for sale only in the state of Nevada, has also proved ineffective for memory enhancement but seems to have some use as a weak antidepressant.

Other possibilities for treating behavioral symptoms include medications for depression, anxiety, agitation, and sleep disturbance. In some cases, major tranquilizer antipsychotic drugs known as butrophones, such as haloperidol (brand name Haldol), seem to have a calming effect on some agitated patients. Other patients become even more agitated, however, especially if the correct dosage is not arrived at with the coop-

---

6. Charles Leroux, "The Silent Epidemic," quoting Jerome Stone, © *Chicago Tribune*, September 1981.

eration of the family and physician. These drugs are used to help the family manage the patient; they are *not* used to treat the illness. However, the fact that haloperidol is a sedative and anticholinergic means that too high a dosage can make memory worse. *The dosage prescribed is crucial.* It is better to start with a smaller dosage and increase gradually until the patient is adequately stabilized. In essence, giving the patient a sedative or minor tranquilizer is a tradeoff since memory problems and confusion may increase as behavior becomes better controlled.

Also, there are serious and chronic effects with prolonged use of major tranquilizers. For example, tardive dyskinesia is a syndrome associated with long-term use of antipsychotic drugs such as phenothiazines, chlorpromazine (Thorazine), trifluoperazine hydrochloride (Stelazine), and prochlorperazine (Compazine) and causes involuntary, rapid, uncontrolled, jerky motor movements and lip smacking.

Many drugs can aggravate cognitive impairment. The behavior of people who take some drugs, such as Proprandol, mimics Alzheimer's symptoms. Other drug offenders that are commonly prescribed for heart disease, hypertension, diabetes, or anxiety are chlorpromazine, bromides, methyldopa, clonidine, phenytoin, quinidine, atropine, phenobarbital, cimetidine, disopyramide, haloperidol, paraldehyde, primidone, and procainamide. The only way to determine if a drug is a factor is to stop the medication for a trial period. The same is true with alcohol. Alcoholics who stop drinking show greatly improved cognition (thinking), unless they have Korsakoff's disease.

Psychostimulants, such as caffeine, have been tried as a treatment approach. While caffeine may pep the person up with energy, it does not improve memory function.

Cognition is also affected by many drugs that are usually not suspect. For example, many older adults commonly take several prescription drugs at the same time. These may be for chronic conditions—for example, a diuretic (water pill) to control high blood pressure, tranquilizers for nervous conditions, sedatives for sleeplessness. In addition, over-the-counter drugs such as aspirin or laxatives may all be taken in the course of a day, and a little wine or a cocktail before dinner may be added. The combination of any or all of these drugs and alcohol or the drugs themselves can be extremely harmful to the memory and thinking processes of the older person.

Ongoing Research

Though the problems of dementing illness were ignored by physicians and scientists for years, the good news is that potentially fruitful research continues and effective treatments are on the horizon.

New research has been aimed at replacing the acetylcholine neurotransmitter substance that helps the brain function in a normal way. At Dartmouth Medical School, pumps implanted surgically in the stomachs of four Alzheimer's patients were used to inject bethanichol chloride, a drug that mimics ACH. The families of three patients reported improvement. The fourth patient remained the same, which, since Alzheimer's disease is progressive, might be considered an improvement. However, this technique is still experimental and not approved as a treatment. Other new research is ongoing with similar drugs that work on the neurotransmitter system.

Neuropeptides, such as vasopressin, have been closely studied. Vasopressin studies are reported as useful in the treatment of elderly patients with mild cognitive impairments. Vasopressin is administered as a nasal inhalant because there has been evidence, although equivocal, that nerve endings sensitive to smell may pick up vasopressin and transport it to the brain, where it acts as a stimulant to improve memory. Evidence as to its effectiveness in reducing the primary symptoms of memory loss has not been satisfactorily demonstrated.

Neurotransmitter precursors, such as choline and lecithin, or agonists, such as physostigmine and arecoline, have also been interesting areas for research. The precursors do not seem to work at all. But physostigmine (in combination with lecithin) in low dosages may temporarily ameliorate the memory disturbances of Alzheimer's disease. Arecoline seems to be able to make memory function better, but there is no practical and effective day-to-day treatment as yet.

The most promising theoretical observation is that the making of acetylcholine in the brain is impaired, but the results of treatment that is based on the cholinergic precursor hypothesis are preliminary and thus far disappointing.

Another theory is that dopamine may play a role in Alzheimer's disease as it does in Parkinson's disease.

Piracetam, a substance that is believed to be an enhancer of brain metabolism, together with choline acetyltransferase (an enzyme found in the brain in neurons that produce and release ACH) have also been researched.

Since choline is the raw material for the synthesis of ACH, could it be that the combination of lecithin, choline, and the agonist physostigmine may also prove to be the most effective treatment since they increase cholinergic function?

What role do blood vessels play in Alzheimer's disease? How the blood carries nutrients and ions such as sodium and potassium to the brain and how it is altered in Alzheimer's disease is the subject of a new research study in Oklahoma. The study will focus on how cells that regulate biochemical activity are processed across the blood brain barrier. It will clarify the role of the decline in blood vessel functioning in the brain due to age and how this may contribute to Alzheimer's disease.

Another research study suggests that the role of enzymes in breaking down protein is important in Alzheimer's disease. The enzyme macropain is being tested. Researchers want to know how macropain attacks specific proteins that are "tagged" by another protein named ubiquitin. Ubiquitin-tagged proteins appear to accumulate in Alzheimer's patients, suggesting that something has gone wrong in the cellular protein breakdown system of the brain.

Researchers in Illinois are investigating the role of corticosteroids in Alzheimer's disease. Corticosteroids are hormones produced by the adrenal glands when there is stress or danger; they stimulate cells to burn energy. In response to excess stress, corticosteroids may accumulate in the hippocampus region of the brain, causing the nerve cells to deplete their energy reserves. The damaged cells may die, affecting memory.

THE MOST PROMISING NEW TREATMENT

Tacrine hydrochloride, formerly known as tetrahydroaminoacridine, or THA, has been found—in a study led by Dr. William K. Summers of UCLA—to be beneficial; it slightly improved intellectual functioning in twelve Alzheimer's patients treated with the drug for three to twenty-six months. The chemical tacrine inhibits an enzyme in the brain, acetylcholine esterase. This enzyme breaks down ACH. The difficulty with the drug is its side effect: liver damage caused by elevated liver enzyme levels. The FDA has not approved marketing tacrine (as Cognex) on a widespread basis.

In an investigation of THA reported in the British journal *Lancet* (27 April 1991), a relatively large sample was studied: eighty-nine patients, of whom nineteen were withdrawn, owing to side effects and five others dropped out for other reasons. These patients received either THA or a placebo for thirteen weeks. After four weeks they were switched to the opposite procedure. Relatively simple tasks showed improvement, there was little change in complex ones. There were no changes in the daily living activities measure. Researchers believe that tacrine can only slow the disease down.

Caution to Caregivers: While tacrine is the most promising new treatment, there is not yet any reason to believe it can do anything beyond slowing the progress of Alzheimer's disease. The question that must be answered is whether noticeable improvement in daily living skills is worth the risk of the drug's side effects.

Participating in Research

At any given time there are many ongoing research studies into new treatments for Alzheimer's disease. Most studies involve giving an experimental drug to a group of patients and monitoring their progress, if any. Caregivers are often faced with the question of whether patients should volunteer for such a study. Participating in research can give a patient early access to a potentially helpful drug, but there is no guarantee that the drug will help more than standard treatments, and there are risks.

As an example, in 1987 the Food and Drug Administration allowed tacrine, or THA, to be given to Alzheimer's patients with life-threatening conditions within rigorous studies. Following reports of limited favorable effects, patients and caregivers requested the drug be made more widely available. A program started in 1992 distributes THA through additional doctors, still on an experimental basis but no longer under the strict guidelines of the original study. Your doctor can call 1-800-7COGNEX to locate a physician participating in the expanded trial.

THA increases the amount of acetylcholine in the brains of patients with Alzheimer's disease, which may reduce memory loss and other symptoms. However, if the treatment is incorrectly monitored, in rare cases patients can suffer severe brain damage. This dilemma encapsulates the primary question raised by any study of new medicines: is the patient's potential reward worth the potential risk?

Who is Eligible?

You should find out the requirements of any study before taking the patient to a diagnostic research center. Most studies require the following conditions to be met:

- The patient has mild to moderate Alzheimer's disease, but is otherwise in good health. Few studies involve patients with severe Alzheimer's.
- The patient has a full-time caregiver. The caregiver attends all of the sessions with the patient, monitors that the drug is taken as required, and helps evaluate any change in the patient's symptoms.
- The patient is not taking any other drugs that could interfere with the results of the study. For instance, this condition excludes people taking heart medication from some of the studies.

Often the patient must pass certain tests at the beginning of the study to be eligible for treatment. Among these tests are a medical history, physical exam, electrocardiogram (EKG), magnetic resonance imaging (MRI), computerized axial tomographic (CAT) scan, urine and blood samples, and a battery of neurophysiological and memory tests. Routine check-ups and further tests are usually also required.

SHOULD WE PARTICIPATE?

The question of whether an Alzheimer's disease patient and his caregiver should participate in a controlled study is one that each family must decide for itself. Some caregivers may want to "leave well enough alone," as one family member put it. Others wish to "leave no stone unturned," trying anything and everything to reclaim the minds of their loved ones. In addition to the primary question of reward and risk, there are many other factors to be weighed in making this decision.

Consider that joining a study may cause stress, both physical and emotional. The patient and caregiver may have to travel, meet new doctors, and change their routine at home. Tests can make a patient anxious. The best judge of how well a patient will respond to the study conditions is the family.

Another drawback of joining a controlled study is that the patient may not be able to try other treatments. Study subjects take on a responsibility not to do things which interfere with the test results.

Some families dislike the idea of letting a relative be a subject of experiments. They fear the patient will be regarded only as a number. In our experience patients are treated kindly by researchers. Caregivers are invited to ask questions and receive as much information about the treatment as is available. They often have the chance to join groups of other caregivers as well.

A few caregivers, when facing the prospect of unproven treatments, prefer to take a more holistic approach to a patient's health. They investigate non-medical approaches: natural sources of lecithin and choline, exercise, and mental stimulation.

Our feeling is that if a patient is in the early stages of Alzheimer's disease, a drug research program might be beneficial. For patients who are in more advanced stages of the illness, it is unlikely that any treatment can reverse it.

It is important to keep a realistic attitude about experimental treatments. They are not "miracle cures." Rather, each is one more step on a scientific journey to finding the causes and remedies for Alzheimer's disease. If you can not or choose not to participate in a medical study, work with patient-advocacy groups to keep research well funded. We will all benefit from finding a cure for this inhumane illness.

Conflicting Interests in Research

In recent years the AIDS epidemic has eclipsed Alzheimer's disease in recognition as a devastating illness that requires funding for research and treatment. AIDS has so far affected a younger population, and AIDS activists have led the way in putting pressure on the government to change health policies. Older Alzheimer's patients and their families contend with the lingering perception that senile dementia is natural and by and large have been less willing to vociferously demand attention. Ironically, at one point in the AIDS illness, the two diseases have parallel symptoms.

Although it is essential that money be available for AIDS research, Alzheimer's disease is an equally slow but no less torturous disease. Rather than have two generations vying with each other over funds, it would benefit us all to allocate adequate money for both AIDS and Alzheimer's research and treatment. Groups devoted to defeating Alzheimer's disease can learn from the AIDS activists. In that way, both the old and the young (who will one day hopefully become old) can share the benefits of medical science and the bond of love.

Research on diseases with certain similarities to Alzheimer's may have important implications, such as the isolation of the gene that transmits Huntington's disease and the study of long-latency infectious agents, which include the structurally unique virus for Creutzfield-Jacob disease, a much rarer condition than Alzheimer's. The Andrus Foundation is studying the major factors in the institutionalization of

Alzheimer's patients, particularly at what point families feel they can no longer cope with the care of the patient because of financial and major behavioral problems such as agitation, wandering, and so on. Educational, drug, behavioral, and diagnostic research is being sponsored by the National Institute on Aging and other agencies.

While there is no one treatment for Alzheimer's disease, the patient's ability to deal with memory loss and the loss of language in the early stages of the illness can be treated.

More monies from the federal government and the private sector continue to be needed nationwide to expand research efforts, including improvements in education and counseling programs for families. In the far future, brain transplants may hold the promise for preventing patients with a diseased brain from slipping into the solitude from which there is no recovery.

Alzheimer's Disease Is a Family Affliction

The Alzheimer's patient requires continuous care, constant attention, and emotional support from the family. At the same time, he also needs protection and help as he becomes increasingly dependent. Caregivers are wise to supplement the patient's care with therapy from a mental health professional and a physician who can judiciously prescribe drugs when the confused patient suffers delusions or severe agitation. The behavioral technique of reality orientation may help the patient maximize his strengths. Although this view is controversial and there is no conclusive research, nurses, psychotherapists, physicians, and family members continue to support their own positive clinical experiences. But what of the caregiver's needs and pressing long-term personal concerns? As the patient's memory fades further away, the caregiver carries many battle scars that remain vivid in his own memory.

In order to provide care for the patient, caregivers must also come to terms with their own confusion, fear, frustration, anger, and embarrassment. Sadly they watch the slow disappearance of those characteristics that made up the unique personality of the afflicted loved one. With guilt they welcome some respite from the burden of loving. They also feel guilty about not being able to do enough for the Alzheimer's patient. Just as the medical profession is limited by its knowledge, caregivers are also limited in what they can reasonably do for their Alzheimer's patients and how they can cope with the stress. However, they are not limited in their capacity for feeling. In the next few chapters we will explore the caregivers' often perplexing feelings.

CHAPTER 5

Denial: Say It Isn't So

No one likes to receive bad news. We don't want to hear that a friend or relative is incurably ill. Perhaps, we tell ourselves, the doctors are mistaken. Aunt Jess is just overtired and will be better after a few good nights' sleep. We resist the news of catastrophe or death. Surely the reports are in error! We refuse to accept an unpleasant truth that threatens us. Our ability to care about others, which gives our lives meaning, also makes us vulnerable when those we care about either hurt or disappoint us. And when they are in danger, we become vulnerable to the pain of loss. In order not to feel that pain, we respond by denying the feeling. The message we give ourselves is "Don't feel."

The first reaction of family members to the death of a relative, especially a sudden or violent death, is frequently "It can't be!" or some variant of "Say it isn't so!" This reaction occurs even when the deceased had been ill for some time, and in circumstances where death might be a reasonable expectation. It is our constant hope that somehow the sick relative will once more pull through the crisis and stay with us a while longer; therefore we deny the reality of his death.

This instant denial is part of the way we adapt ourselves to ideas and events too horrible to comprehend all at once. By greeting the news of death or disaster with "No, it can't be true!" we are keeping the impact of the event and its implications at arm's length. We're giving our minds and emotions a chance to adjust, bit by bit, to the new information that might otherwise overwhelm us.

Yet, over time, what can't be gives way to what could be, to what might be, to certainty. In this process, our defense mechanism of denial has helped us to disengage from our feelings, to take distance from the horrible events, and finally to dull and ultimately deaden our emotions. Thus denial protects us from the shock of unwelcome news and helps us control the way we finally receive and accept the facts.

When you ignore the fact that your relative has a problem with memory loss, this form of denial may have dangerous consequences for the Alzheimer's patient, and sometimes for you as well. For example, allowing a memory-impaired person to continue driving the car because he still has physical driving skills may jeopardize his safety as well as that of passengers and others if his judgment has been impaired.

While short-term denial, such as a response of disbelief to a sudden shock or catastrophe, may be a way-station in the process of accepting and dealing with the crisis, denial that persists makes useful action more difficult, if not impossible.

MRS. HARTMAN: "My husband ran his own wholesale agent's business, and even after he was diagnosed as having Alzheimer's disease, he continued with his work, writing orders, sending samples, and verifying shipments. Other people who had relatives afflicted with Alzheimer's disease were amazed—so often it is the ability to work with numbers and details that goes first. They considered me—and my husband—very fortunate. And so did I.

"But it wasn't true. Oh, he got on the phone every day and talked to his customers, and he took orders, just as he always had, so I thought everything was fine. He acted as if everything was fine . . . normal, just like always. But while I thought he was running his business, he was getting everything all mixed up! He was forgetting to stuff the samples into the envelopes, or sending the wrong orders, or he would get lost on the way to the post office and never send anything at all! He acted as if everything was just the same, and I didn't pay enough attention to all these clues because I didn't want to believe the situation was that bad."

47

People who have been deceived in this way are likely to feel frustrated and angry at the patient. It is difficult to realize that the deception was a by-product of the patient's own denial of his worsening condition, and that he was not aware of either the reasons for his actions or their effects. Also, in denying that her husband had become as sick as he actually was, Mrs. Hartman was not willfully ignoring his condition. But it was a relief for her to believe that he was still able to function, since his seeming competence absolved her of the obligation to face the consequences of her husband's inevitable deterioration.

In psychological terms, denial is a defense mechanism in which the person does not admit to himself consciously that painful facts exist. He continues to behave as if he has no problems and in ways that seem comfortable and reassuring to him. But at the same time, this behavior prevents him from having real needs met. This can have serious repercussions in his own life and in the lives of other people. Denying a problem won't make it go away; indeed, it can make the situation worse.

Mr. Hartman, who carried on with his business, and his wife were unable to recognize that recent-memory loss had made him incapable of conducting his daily affairs successfully. Consequently, he was also deprived of the memory aids and confidence builders that are used to ease and support the daily life of an early stage Alzheimer's patient whose condition has been acknowledged and accepted. Perhaps most unfortunately, his impaired abilities actually damaged the strength of the business and undermined the couple's future financial security.

Patients who are in the very early stages of Alzheimer's disease or other similar conditions may worry about their failing powers and sometimes share their concerns with spouses and children. Unfortunately, those who listen to these worries often feel the need to deny the reality of what their afflicted relative is trying to tell them. They respond with: "I don't think you should worry. Remember, you're not as young as you used to be. So maybe you're slowing down a little! You still seem just fine to me." Or, "You know, Dad, you really ought to get more organized. Why don't you make a list before you go to the store? Haven't you got a calculator to check your bank balance with? Well, don't worry, I'll get you one for your birthday."

Unconscious Denial

Often we do not recognize changes that occur in our older family members and therefore ignore what could be early warning signals. Mrs. Grant always handled the budget and paid the bills. She was a genius at switching the money from one account to another just in time to cover the checks that she'd already written. Even when the Grants spent more money than they could afford, she always managed to keep the family solvent.

It took Mr. Grant a long time to learn that anything was wrong with the way his wife was handling the finances. This was partly because he expected their family pattern to be maintained; but it was also because he didn't want to handle the bill paying, a job he considered boring and time-consuming and one that he was happy to relinquish to his wife. He may not even have remembered receiving a "friendly letter" from a credit department a few weeks earlier. He simply asked his wife, "By the way, did you pay them?" and when she said yes, dismissed the matter. When he finally discovered the scope of the problem, he was initially outraged and then alarmed by his wife's continuing to profess ignorance or denying the reality with which he confronted her.

By not paying more attention to the family bill paying at the earliest signs that something was going wrong, Mr. Grant was unconsciously participating in the denial. Family members often do this when the memory-impaired relative complains about a loss of function. Sometimes this denial of the elderly person's concern takes a hostile form. "Mom, there's nothing wrong with you that wouldn't be fine if you'd just go out and make some friends. Since Dad died you just sit around and your only social outlet is talking to me." Or: "You 'forget' on purpose and you're just trying to get me to pay more attention to you. There's nothing else wrong with you." Or: "What's the matter with you, anyway? How many times do I have to answer the same question? I told you already, you just don't listen. You don't need to go to a doctor, you just need to pay more attention when people are talking to you!"

Husbands and wives sometimes unintentionally collaborate in failing to recognize the symptoms that suggest there is something wrong with a spouse for several reasons. Often they are so close to one another that they don't register small changes in mental functioning; they are afraid to contemplate traumatic changes that would take place in their lives in the case of a catastrophic illness; they are also subject to what psycho-analysts refer to as *egoïsme à deux*—the need to be like each other and to cooperate with each other, even in terms of denying reality.

The family's denials can persist until the sufferer's actions become too bizarre to be ignored. By the time a diagnosis is finally made, it may be too late for an orderly transfer of the patient's assets, the securing of a power of attorney, and all the other protections of financial security for the unafflicted spouse or children. In such cases the family's denial of the patient's illness prevents real needs from being met.

For the family of the patient who has been diagnosed as having Alzheimer's disease, the patient's upsetting behaviors are only part of the problem. The healthy family members must be careful not to deny the troubling reality of the nature and progress of the illness.

It is not always clear whether we should tell the patient the facts about the condition. Should we tell the impaired person he has an illness that interferes with memory? Do we really want to admit to ourselves that this is the case? Don't we want to protect our loved ones from the cruelty of that information? "You're losing your memory. It won't come back." Sometimes it might—most of the time it won't.

MRS. VALERIE DUMONT: "My problem is trying to give reassurances to my husband that his condition has been stabilized. I'm aware of the severity of the condition. I went to a neurologist who diagnosed him as having Alzheimer's disease. As yet, according to the doctor, there's been no breakthrough in medical knowledge that could reverse the situation. He said that the only thing you can hope for is that he will reach a plateau and stabilize at that point.

"Well, so far he has not reached that plateau, but I have to keep telling my husband that it won't get any worse. It's very difficult, because it's so obvious to me, it must be obvious to him, too, that he is declining. Am I doing the right thing? Am I doing the wrong thing?

"I always tell him, 'I'm going to tell you the truth!' But I'm not telling him the truth! I keep giving him reassurance by telling him I sense that it probably has reached that plateau. I can't give him any evidence of it because I know it is not so. But I feel that if I don't encourage him, it's going to have an adverse effect on him. I'm fearful of what the consequences might be . . . you know, his mother was hopelessly senile at the end. Yet in my heart I can't say that I ever think he's going to be like his mother."

No one can tell Valerie Dumont whether she is doing the right thing or the wrong thing in falsely reassuring her husband that his condition has stabilized. But she may, despite her protests, be trying to deny to herself the fact that her husband's condition is worsening when she says, "In my heart I can't say that I ever think he's going to be like his mother." In trying to assure her husband, she may be helping him, and herself as well, to deny the reality of his condition. She shows some awareness of her own defense mechanism when she adds:

"What I want is to give him comfort. And of course, when I think about it, I realize that it's giving me greater comfort to believe that his condition has stabilized. Otherwise the pain, the anguish, is too much. After all, without his memory, what will happen to our relationship?"

Indeed, when memory fades, so do the treasured moments of love, joy, and intimacy, as well as sorrow, pain, and anger. Without memory, can there be love? The constancy of a formerly caring person can be lost in the penultimate moments of this treacherous disease. Yet the caregiver's memory remains. It is a bond of love that enables the caregiver to sacrifice and to suffer, while ironically, the memory of the victim of Alzheimer's disease fades and is finally lost.

"No, it cannot be true," is the initial response of denial when a relative is told that a loved one has Alzheimer's disease.

MR. SANDS: "I can't believe that my mother will ever disintegrate like that. Because I know that I would not be able to take it—I couldn't. Look

51

at her, just look at her! She's the picture of health! How can you believe that something's wrong with her mentally!"

Family members who cannot face the pain of chronic illness and the nearness of death have to put away these thoughts in order to continue the pursuit of their everyday lives. After such shocking news, denial is a defense that acts as a buffer, allowing the family members to collect themselves.

MRS. EDMONDS: "We just learned that my husband has this disease called senile dementia. He's still in the early stages, and I'm optimistic. I'm not sure I want to hear about the problems he will have in the later stages. I don't want to hear anything worse."

The continual search for medications and a variety of treatments for the Alzheimer's patient may be an example of denial by the caregivers, but it is also an example of the great devotion that family members have for their memory-impaired relatives.

MR. ISAACS: "I'm disgusted with the whole medical profession. These doctors, they really don't know very much, whatever they tell you. My mother has some strange habits—she keeps forgetting which day of the week it is, and she sometimes gets up in the middle of the night and gets dressed to go shopping. I couldn't figure out why she would do that. Finally, it began to bother me so much that I took her to a psychiatrist. He said he really couldn't find very much wrong with her and said she's just a little senile. So I took her to a neurologist. He said that she had brain cells that were damaged, but he couldn't prescribe anything. So I took her to a mnemonist—a memory specialist—who worked with her for several months, giving her safety pins to pin notes on her lapel. Before we were done with her—the memory specialist—Mother had notes on every article of clothing. Then we heard about a health foods advocate who said that she could cure forgetfulness with massive doses of lecithin. So I bought the lecithin and Mother took it twice a day, every day, for a year. I took it, too—it was terrible-tasting stuff. And while she didn't seem to be getting any more weird in her behavior, the same problems were still there. Now I've heard about this experimental drug program, which I hope to enroll her in next week."

However, even after the family has exhausted all of the physicians' resources (which, unfortunately, are few) and the researchers' drugs (which are, equally unfortunately, not very effective), the search for a drug that will restore their relatives' memory may continue. This can be a form of denial of the illness.

While "hope springs eternal in the human breast," and while we must feel a sense of hopefulness in order to go on living, expending emotional and physical energies and financial resources is, beyond a certain point, a form of denial.

Acknowledging the Problem

It is difficult to acknowledge that the behavior of someone you love has changed radically. However, when that person shows diminished vitality, is less capable than before, has fewer internal controls, is lacking in independent activity, and becomes more irritable, increasingly volatile, and considerably more forgetful than before, you will have difficulty ignoring the evidence of your own daily experience. An accumulation of incidents will bring you to the point where you must acknowledge that something terrible is happening to the relative or friend you care about. After a diagnosis is made, you will find yourself forced to consider the possibility that he may not recover. The probability is that he will become unable to do things for himself, and you may be the one who must take over the major burden of caregiving.

The moment of this realization can be very frightening. Most people feel dazed, immobilized, and disbelieving: "What's going to happen? What will I do? What can I do?" Some people cover over their fears of the unknown and keep right on going. "We'll do as much as we can for as long as we can. It will be all right."

Whatever your response to this major change in your life, very likely nothing in your past has prepared you for an experience of this magnitude. Many people have these feelings as they assume the role of caregiver to a patient with Alzheimer's disease. What is important to keep in mind is that you have successfully managed to meet previous challenges in your life. You can draw on your inner strengths to master this challenge as well. It is more fruitful for you to acknowledge the illness and to accept the fact that while there is really nothing that can be done to reverse the condition, you can still care for the person, make him as comfortable as possible, and show him kindness and affection. Without this acceptance, your much-needed resources will be drained away.

Some of the best and most helpful advice is the simplest: take one day at a time. It is almost impossible to anticipate what might happen next in the life of a person who has a memory-impairing disease, and it may often be better not to try. Taking life one day at a time is not only practical advice; it may realistically be the most constructive thing you can do.

While your behavior will benefit from a "one day at a time" philosophy, your feelings about your relative's memory loss will vary. You will experience fear of the unknown course of the illness; sadness as you remember and mourn a relationship that will never be the same; anger that you have been singled out for this trial; despair when you doubt your ability to cope; guilt when you worry that you haven't done everything for the impaired person, or when you feel love slipping away under the stress of daily frustrations; resentment when this person fails to respond to you in loving ways that you've grown accustomed to expect.

Your feelings will influence the way you deal with your patient, the other members of your family, and those people in the medical and helping professions who try to assist you with your patient's various needs. Sometimes these feelings may cause you extreme discomfort. Remember at such times that there aren't any "shoulds" or "should nots" when it comes to your feelings. Someone may say to you, "At your age, you shouldn't be feeling this way." Why not? You're entitled to your feelings, whatever they may be. Don't let anyone tell you that your feelings are "wrong." Feelings are neither right nor wrong, they just are.

What is most important is that you try to understand your own feelings and those of others. For example, if every time your spouse goes off into a room by himself and closes the door you feel rejected, that feeling may influence ont only the way you behave toward him, but also the way you behave toward yourself (telling yourself it must be something you said or did that's making him push you away). He may tell you that it's wrong for you to feel rejected when he closes the door. Let him know that when he does that, it makes you feel isolated and alone. If you understand why you're feeling rejected, and that the way you behave results from these feelings, this understanding can help you to cope better, both with the feelings themselves and with everyday life.

Very often we don't take the time and trouble to understand why we're feeling a certain way. We are so busily engaged in everyday living and work that we don't take the time to wonder: Why did I get so angry? What makes me feel so embarrassed? Can I do something for myself so that I don't feel so helpless? It is helpful to rid ourselves of angry feelings so that we can be in touch with more loving feelings. If we don't explore the reasons for our negative reactions to people and to situations, we will repeat these same reactions over and over again. Think about why you feel the way you do. Chances are that the next time a similar situation arises, you will know what provoked your anger earlier, and you can then behave in a more positive way.

Much of our behavior, including our responses to our feelings, is automatic. Flying off the handle when your relative repeats words or behaves childishly is a response that won't change until you understand what that behavior means to you. We must consciously act to change a negative behavior. No doubt, easier said than done—but not impossible.

In order to change habitual ways of thinking and feeling, it is important to have some insight into ourselves. Sometimes the change in behavior can come first. For example, you could say that you're never going to eat so much, or take another drink again, or get so mad again, and stick to it. But you would be much more likely to stick to it if you understood what feelings provoke the overeating, excess drinking, or uncontrolled anger.

Mutual Support Groups

In the last few years, a remarkable change has occurred in the experience of families who care for victims of Alzheimer's disease and similar memory-impairing illnesses: they have discovered each other and come together for mutual support and encouragement. The shame and isolation that formerly kept families from sharing their burden has given way to a desire for more public information, more research, and of equal importance, mutual support in confronting the problems of memory impairment in those we love and in dealing with our feelings about being caregivers. The Alzheimer's Disease and Related Disorders Association, founded in 1979, helps people around the country establish support groups and share medical and scientific information.

In a support group, when you hear other families of Alzheimer's victims who have similar problems, you may be able to understand your own feelings, both toward your memory-impaired relative and about yourself. You will be able to give and to receive support and strength. You might gain enough insight to be able to change your situation and relieve yourself of some of your burden.

In the following pages, we will talk about some of the feelings caregivers have as they live with and care for their memory-impaired relatives and friends. These caregivers are in situations similar to the one in which you now find yourself. They have dealt with forgetfulness, catastrophic reactions (temper tantrums), confusions of word and thought, and physical and emotional problems in their loved ones. They have acknowledged their own fears, despair, frustrations, and pain and have wrestled with the difficult practical questions of money, household safety, and the painful decision of when or whether to put a declining, frail spouse or parent in a nursing home. By learning how others have faced the emotional impact of caring for an Alzheimer's patient, you can gain strength and confidence in dealing with these same emotions and decisions.

CHAPTER 6

Anger:
The Perplexing Emotion

Ms. ZABRISKI: "My uncle was always very sweet and nice. But when he came to live with us I had to give up my job to stay home with him. That made me angry, and I yelled at him a lot. Even while I was yelling, I thought, 'Oh, this is terrible, he's sick, he's fragile.' And then he'd get mad at me. One day he was so furious he left the house, slamming the door—something he'd never done before—and disappeared. We had to search the whole neighborhood for him. He scared me to death when he got lost like that. So I never yelled at him again."

Ms. MCKAY: "I took my sister shopping with me when I went to the supermarket, as I usually do. And when we were leaving the market, I noticed that she was chewing gum. She's not usually a gum chewer. So I asked her, 'Where did you get that gum?' And she pointed, 'In there.' She'd taken it, simply because she wanted it—like shoplifting! Well, I was so furious! I grabbed the rest of the pack from her, and I threw it down, and I yelled at her: 'You're not supposed to do that; you shouldn't have that!' What could I do? I was too ashamed to go back into the store and return it—too embarrassed."

Anger, shame, embarrassment, fear—almost everyone who lives with a person whose memory is impaired is familiar with these feelings.

People with memory loss often behave in bizarre or unexpected ways that frustrate, exhaust, and embarrass us.

These behaviors make us feel annoyance, impatience, irritation, resentment, fury, and rage, all of which belong to the range of feelings known as anger. As family members encounter continual memory failures on the part of their relative, the initial denial of the patient's illness is replaced by a variety of feelings such as grief, sorrow, upset—and anger.

Anger is a very human reaction to frustration, disappointment, and grief. We have a right to our feelings, and appropriate anger, like fear, is a normal reaction. It is a basic emotion that helps us to survive. Feeling angry when we are cheated, lied to, or taken advantage of, or when we are disappointed in the behavior of others, helps protect us from the pain of experiencing ourselves as helpless, vulnerable creatures.

Healthy people feel anger many times in their lives. The ability to feel anger tells us that we care about someone or something deeply enough to feel discomfort and to verbalize our displeasure. For each of us, angry feelings conjure up different anecdotes and situations, varied experiences and responses.

Why Does She Do Those Embarrassing Things?

Loss of memory, particularly in the case of patients with Alzheimer's disease, is neither orderly nor selective. Therefore patients can lose from their memories any information or behavior that has been learned. Such patients can forget how to tell time or the name of a loved one or wife. Inappropriate behavior such as shoplifting may result from a loss of impulse control.

From our earliest childhood we have been taught how to behave in society. We learned the mores of the groups we belong to, the laws and how to live within them, and how to act in public places. We also learned to rely upon the same knowledge in others.

People who break the various social codes (whether they do so intentionally, or whether, like the victim of Alzheimer's disease, they have forgotten those codes) are mistrusted, avoided, scorned, and criticized.

This disapproval is embarrassing to other family members when they feel that the confused patient's behavior is a reflection on them.

The woman who helped herself to the chewing gum had simply forgotten the whole process of selecting an item and paying for it. She saw the gum, she wanted it, and acting on impulse, she took it. Ms. McKay, on the other hand, whose memory is intact and who therefore knows this aspect of society's rules, was terribly embarrassed at the thought of what her neighbors and the store manager would say about her forgetful sister's behavior. Ms. McKay was ashamed that her sister had done such a thing and felt responsible, but her initial reaction was irritation at her sister for having caused her this embarrassment.

Even before we understood the demands of group living, we were learning patterns of everyday behavior, which include such mundane activities as brushing our teeth, tying shoelaces, taking a shower, telling time, and using the toilet, daily habits that we have practiced since we were children. Most of these seemingly simple habits are in fact complicated sequences of behavior that have become an automatic part of our everyday lives. We rarely think about these activities as we engage in them, but they are vital to our ability to function as independent adults. The patient's loss of memory for such activities, resulting in his need for constant reminders and assistance, is one of the major sources of irritation, frustration, and anger for immediate family members who are caregivers to the impaired person.

Ms. Lovett: "I have to bathe and shave and dress him. And the worst thing is to have to clean his mouth. If you have any sense of personal hygiene, the mouth is the dirtiest part of the body! God bless dentists! I don't know how they can stand to work in our mouths!"

Mr. Gettinger: "My wife will put her pajamas on over her underwear. I have to tell her she's got to take her underwear off. She never changes her underwear or her clothes. I have to do it for her. She won't take a shower. I have to make her do it. Then we both get upset."

Ms. Corcoran: "The bathroom's another problem. When he has to go to the bathroom, he can't tell me whether he has to sit or stand. If he tries to sit when he has to urinate, his penis gets all cockeyed. I never know where the urine is going to end up. It's so undignified. I feel resentful. And the frustration—I'm so agitated, there are days when I could just let go and let somebody have it. Why do I feel so indignant— and afterwards, so guilty?"

In addition to learning codes of social behavior and developing personal habits, we also learned how to absorb information. In school we studied history, geography, languages, and mathematics and the techniques for manipulating facts and numbers. Besides paying attention to and remembering what we have read, we learned to pay attention to what others tell us and to remember what they say.

Often, when someone close to us develops Alzheimer's disease, the first observable symptom is forgetfulness of his own actions or of instructions from others. In the early stages of the disease, sufferers tend to mislay familiar objects like eyeglasses and car keys and to forget what they are told.

As the person's memory loss increases, he may forget to run errands or to fulfill special requests. You may find yourself reacting with irritation and scorn to his forgetfulness: "Where did you put the darn car keys this time?"

"Dammit, honey, the last thing I said before we left the house was, 'Don't forget to pick up the bills, because we want to mail them on our way so we won't be charged interest for late payments.' You irritate me when you ignore me like that . . . I don't think you ever listen to me!"

"What's the matter with you? I told you last week to take my coat to the cleaners. Do you want me to go out looking like a bum? I'll bet you didn't get my coat cleaned on purpose, just to bug me."

It may seem to the healthy spouse or child that the forgetful family member is not forgetful at all, but willfully ignoring his desires. The patient's forgetfulness may seem to reflect on the caregiver's competence as well: "How can you go out dressed like that, with a checkered shirt and a striped jacket? The neighbors will think I don't pay any attention to you, to let you go out of the house that way. I'll be so embarrassed!"

As memory losses increase, other aspects of behavior are affected. A patient may ask the same question over and over again but be unable to remember your answer. The very repetition of the question is provocative and can be maddening.

Mr. Dayton: "You get to a certain point where you feel like you've been pushed beyond endurance. Last week, my aunt lost her watch. The band is too large now, so it slipped off her arm. You go over it what seems like a hundred times: 'It's here somewhere, don't be upset. We're going to find it.' And then you find that the quiet, rational talk is just not getting through, because two minutes later she asks: 'Where's my watch?' You go through all this, and it happens with so many different things, that you eventually get to the point where your good nature and a smile won't sustain you."

Ms. Jordan: "I make dinner for us every night. He can still feed himself, and he eats everything I set in front of him. So last night I made a nice pot roast, vegetables, gravy, a real feast. I cleaned up, washed the pots, and just as I was putting away the plates, he asked me, 'What am I going to eat for dinner tonight?' I felt so incensed that I almost threw the plates at him!"

Mr. Meeker: "My brother and I have always made an occasion of going out to eat together. We'd have dinner at a restaurant about once a month. It was our way of staying together. But lately it's torture for me. Last week when we were out, he was slurping his food and drooling on his necktie, and I was mortified. But the worst! The worst was when dinner was over. All of a sudden, with no warning, he pulled out his dentures and began to swish them around in his coffee cup! I could have died right there on the spot. I was so mortified that I became furious with him."

Sometimes we become exasperated because we are ashamed of our relative's behavior and embarrassed at having to endure the stares of friends and strangers. The first thought is, "Why is he behaving like this?" followed, perhaps, by "How could he do this to me?" These reactions are spontaneous, despite the fact that we know our relative has lost the ability to control his own behavior and can't remember social etiquette.

When your relative's symptoms first appeared, it's not surprising that you assumed he still was able to use his memory and manage his own actions. It sometimes takes a while before you realize that this is the third or fourth time the coat didn't get to the cleaners; that the eyeglasses are "lost" a dozen times a day; that notes and frequent reminders don't seem to have an impact.

An accumulation of such experiences may make the irritated husband or wife suspect that something more serious than simple forgetfulness is happening. There weren't enough arguments recently to blame spitefulness for the oversights and neglected errands. Hanging up a key rack hasn't kept the keys from getting lost.

But inflammatory feelings toward your forgetful family member may ensue; they may even increase. At the moment that you, as the husband, wife, or child of a forgetful spouse or parent begin to consider the possibility that your relative has become severely ill, your shock, grief, and fear may turn to anger. Often, anger is a more comfortable response to your fear of the unknown disease or its uncharted course. We do tend to become angry when we feel frightened, hurt, or threatened. Healthy family members feel extremely vulnerable when they discover the nature of their relative's illness.

The degree of vulnerability that you and other family members feel usually depends on the type of relationship that existed between you and the patient prior to the onset of the illness. If, for example, a wife has been completely dependent on her husband to take care of all the family financial matters, she may find that paying bills and managing a checkbook are very threatening activities for her. Decision making may tax her former view of herself as being dependent and needing to be taken care of.

Likewise, men who have depended totally upon their wives to maintain the household, plan and prepare meals, choose their friends, and organize the entertainment may also be at a loss as to how to care for a sick wife and manage their domestic affairs.

The feeling of vulnerability may make the caregiver feel bitterness toward the impaired spouse for having "deserted" him or her, especially as the two are approaching old age. Plans to retire and spend the remaining years living comfortably and companionably together are foiled. Perhaps they intended to do many things that were postponed for one reason or another. Now the healthy relative is cut off from the person who had been depended upon for warmth, physical comfort, emotional understanding, sex, and companionship. The long-awaited fulfillment of the poet's lines—"Grow old along with me! The best is yet to be"—has been thwarted by a chronic illness. Becoming upset and even enraged under these circumstances is a reaction to the tremendous frustration in the face of these life events.

The Patient Isn't the Only Problem

All of us experience anxieties and tensions to some degree or other. The caregivers of Alzheimer's patients, in particular, live not only with the daily pressures and tensions of ordinary living, but also with the constant intensity of an enormous responsibility. Caregivers suffer anxieties about their own mental and physical health. They wonder whether they, too, will become victims of Alzheimer's disease, and they worry about the possible loss of the loved one. These emotions can tax the healthiest human psyche.

Along with the constant drain we face from our own anxieties and tensions, we frequently find ourselves irritated with physicians who may not be able to give us concrete information about the course of the illness. We may feel abandoned and even cheated when professional people don't have all the answers and cannot give us advice about how to handle the patient's behavior.

Physicians, because they often know little about this disease and how it affects their patients, are the first targets of families' resentment: the doctors don't know what tests to give, they are uncertain about what drugs to prescribe, they spend too little time with the families, and they charge too much money.

Ms. GILHOOLEY: "I really am angry at the medical community! There's so much mouthing off about what is being done in the field, and in the area of research, but I don't see that anything concrete is really being done to help my cousin! These people in medicine, they say they're working on it, and they're doing the best they can, and they've got this program and that service. Then, when I try to get more specific and ask about their results, the tune is, 'The drugs are merely experimental. We have no definitive results yet.' It's so frustrating!"

MR. MARTIN: "Although my wife was diagnosed as having Alzheimer's disease over two years ago, up until the last year or so she was still functioning fairly well. As an accountant, until last year she still did occasional assignments. But we have been spending the winters in Florida for many years, so last winter I asked the doctor, since she wasn't in quite as good shape as she had been, if he thought we should still go to Florida. He told us to go because she'd be better off in a warmer climate.

"Well, he was absolutely wrong. In Florida, she woke up in the middle of the night and started beating on the furniture. I called my doctor long distance, rather than taking my wife to an unfamiliar doctor in Florida, because I figured he knew her history and her condition. My doctor prescribed a tranquilizer that had an absolutely disastrous effect on my wife. She became rigid. We had to take her to the emergency room of the hospital. They gave her a shot and told us to let her relax at home until the drug wore off. It was a horrible experience; it made me furious with my doctor!"

Caregivers—and sometimes physicians as well—must learn from trial and error which drugs are helpful to the patient with Alzheimer's disease and which are not. Drugs sometimes have adverse and unexpected effects on individuals. Family members feel irritated and angry when a professional person does not act in the best interest of their patients. Although we may tend to treat him as such, a physician is not a god. He may or may not have knowledge about the illness or be able to help the family. If he can accept his own limitations, he will advise the family to seek another medical consultation and, one hopes, will recommend a neurologist or other colleague who can be more helpful to the patient. At the very least, the physician should be able to suggest other paths for the family to follow.

Understanding and Managing Anger

Sometimes, the frustration and anger that you feel about another aspect of your life can be carried over into your relationship with the memory-impaired person. Anger tends to be visited on the person who has the fewest available defenses.

Mr. Kucera: "I had a punching match with my brother last week. I'm 82 and he's nearly 90, so it wasn't exactly Dempsey and Willard. But he kept asking me the same question over and over again, and I got annoyed. I know why I punched him . . . it actually had nothing to do with him. I was infuriated with my wife. She'd been nagging me the whole morning long about this bill and that expense, and how much we're contributing to my brother George. It was just like when the kids were small, and she would scold and nag at me. Those were the times when I couldn't stand the racket that the children were making, and I would yell at them and shut them up in their rooms for punishment, or spank them. Of course it was really her, not them, that I wanted to spank.

"Today I went back to my brother to apologize, I felt so guilty. Even though he didn't remember, I said I was sorry. It made me feel better."

Sometimes we project our anger onto our environment and become infuriated with doctors and other professionals or vent our rage on an object, such as a car, when we are irritated with ourselves. Often, as in Mr. Kucera's case, some action of the patient provokes us, and it is the patient at whom we tend to direct our wrath. At the moment an upsetting incident occurs, our intellectual understanding that the memory-impaired patient is not actually responsible for his behavior disappears. All we can feel is our own irritation and perhaps rage. At that point, in

65

response to our fury, we may lash out at the person who caused our shame and embarrassment.

Sometimes our response is overt or obvious, and we shout or pound the table. We might be shaking with rage from head to toe, and there are times when we may grab and shake the offending relative.

Of course, we don't always ventilate our anger by shouting or by becoming physically violent. Irritation and annoyance can also be expressed by glowering frowns, leers, sulking, pouting, snide or nasty comments, sick jokes, and other kinds of visual and verbal hostility. For example, one sadistic husband, frustrated with his wife's loss of skills and dismayed at having to assume most of the household chores, would challenge her whenever she asked if she could help him around the house. Although she had lost the ability to read or write, when she offered to help he would tell her to make out the shopping list. Since he knew that the task was impossible for her, this suggestion was his way of venting his anger at her for the discomfort she was causing him. It certainly would have been more helpful and appropriate for him to suggest that she peel vegetables or dry the dishes, tasks she might have been able to handle more comfortably.

Equally potent, but more subtle and disguised, is "passive" anger. A wife who seems to bury her resentment, to remain calm and loving no matter what the provocation, may later "forget" to give her husband his medication on time. She would never forget something so important on purpose, and the oversight is not, in fact, intentional or conscious, but it may have the same damaging consequences as a physical blow. Or perhaps she will "forget" to take her spouse to the bathroom and later scold him for having an "accident." Other expressions of passive anger on the part of the caregiver may include failing to express any tenderness or concern, ignoring the spouse or parent or not paying attention to his needs, or inadvertently leaving an object where the impaired person might easily collide with it and be hurt.

The emotion of anger is the opposite of love. Indeed, it is a destroyer of love and respect in human relationships; therefore, cultural and family pressures teach us to repress our anger. Yet, when our angry feelings are given free expression, the air is cleared for the exchange of loving feelings that have been blocked by unexpressed emotion. No one can deny our right to feel anger, but how our anger is expressed is of utmost importance in the struggle to feel compassion and empathy toward the person who is ill.

Furthermore, when anger is repressed it inevitably produces anxiety, a component of fear. While fear is a reaction to a specific stimulus, anxiety is an unfocused sense of fearfulness. Emotional distress about some unknown future danger overtakes us. Often, the anxiety is described as "free floating"—we do not know the source. Caregivers' anxieties may also be reflected by the patient's behavior; see Chapter 9 for more information on family members' common fears.

As the major caregiver, you may become so frightened of your rage that you cringe from expressing it toward anyone. Fearful of losing control, you may then internalize the anger, which later reappears as self-destructive behavior. Compulsive types of self-destructive behavior patterns include overeating, drinking to excess, and the use of habit-forming drugs such as cocaine or tranquilizers. In other forms of self-flagellation, caregivers may develop physical symptoms, including headaches, stomach aches or backaches, or psychosomatic ailments such as ulcers or colitis. Masochistic blaming of oneself for the patient's illness is another form of self-destructive behavior.

It is important to understand that aggression and rage (an extreme form of aggression) are reactions to the frustration we feel when we are disappointed in a loved one and in ourselves. Repressed anger tends to reappear as anxiety and other upsetting feelings. Thus we must realize that it is equally important for children as well as adults who live with (or near) a relative who has Alzheimer's disease to express their negative feelings verbally. The child's need to talk things out is as great as the adult's. For example, the child may be irritated by the hyperactive behavior of his grandmother who has Alzheimer's disease if she interferes with his play. The child may be embarrassed by a memory-impaired grandfather who calls him home for supper, even though supper was over an hour ago. Owing to the limitations of space, the ailing adult may be forced to share the child's room, thus intruding on and violating the child's privacy and freedom.

Children and adults who feel ashamed, humiliated, or ignored often express their anger through outbursts of temper, provoked by the difficulties and frustrations of living with an Alzheimer's patient. Some people may react as soon as the Alzheimer's patient begins repeating a phrase or in some other way indicating his helplessness.

The feelings of anger that are elicited by the frustration of such circumstances are perfectly understandable. But acting out the anger is another matter. Not only is your outburst likely to alarm or confuse your patient; the guilt you feel when the storm is over may well contribute to further resentment.

Dealing with Frustration

Controlling one's temper and developing more patience are common difficulties for caregivers and their children. Rather than popping a tranquilizer into your mouth to relieve your tension, find an outlet for your frustration. Discussing your feelings with other family members or a close friend can be soothing. The feeling that someone understands you and what you are going through can be very comforting.

You may be able to minimize your frustration by releasing it physically through an activity such as walking, running, engaging in a sport, vigorous housework, or chopping wood. Or you may find release in meditation and relaxation techniques such as the following:

Imagine a scene that is especially peaceful to you, a place where you usually feel relaxed and calm. Take a few deep breaths and try to visualize that serene and pacific scene. This technique may effectively calm you down in a few moments when you become impatient or feel that you are about to explode. It's like "counting to ten" with a visual image. As you discover that you can control yourself, your sense of self-confidence will increase and your feelings of self-esteem will rise.

Another relaxation exercise, for which you will need a quiet corner and about fifteen minutes without interruption, entails kicking off your shoes, closing your eyes, and making your mind a blank screen. Take yourself on a guided fantasy. Have a minivacation in your favorite place—perhaps it's a mountain glade or a sandy beach. Feel the cool wind in your hair or the warm water covering your feet. Listen to the whisper of the breeze in the pines or palm trees. You have a tall cool drink in your hand. You are lying down, perfectly relaxed. Think about how free and wonderful you feel. Your whole body is relaxed; each bone and muscle is loose; you are feeling oh, so very good. Remain that way for at least fifteen minutes. When you get up, you will feel as refreshed as if you had had a relaxing sleep. Take yourself "away" for a few moments every day. It will relieve some of the intense feeling of burden and loss that you experience daily and will help to restore and "re-create" yourself.

Feeling renewed in this fashion will help you to remain calm and loving even in those difficult situations when your relative's repetitive and hyperactive behavior tries your patience or some bizarre action embarrasses you.

Even so, there are moments when the forbearance, the understanding, and the compassion that you have tried to maintain desert you, and again you may react to your relative's behavior with a growl or an inflamed, unkind outburst. As a result, seeing his relative and caregiver so worked up may increase the confusion and agitation of the patient.

MS. BATES: "My brother and I were very close . . . we were almost like twins when we were small, and even after we grew up we wanted to be together. So after we got married, we stayed in the same town we'd grown up in, and we bought houses next door to each other. My brother Sammy is a very likable fellow. At least he was until he got sick. Now I'm not so sure.

"We raised our kids together and we lived alongside each other all this time. Sammy's wife, my sister-in-law, died pretty young and it wasn't long after Sammy's kids left home that he moved in with us. In some ways, that was the best time of my life, to have both John and Sammy there. Sammy fixed things when John was too busy; he did special favors for me, and when John died four years ago, I leaned on him completely. I don't think I could have survived the experience without him.

"Then he started getting forgetful. He'd take the car out and forget to put the keys back on the shelf. I'd send him to the store for milk—just milk—and he'd forget it. Or sometimes he'd go twice and we'd have enough milk for a month!

"He began to have trouble on his job, too. He was an accountant, and he would visit various companies and check their books. It got so he was having a lot of trouble checking the books. Since he was a senior man in the firm, he always took an assistant with him when he visited a client. The assistant did all the arithmetic that Sammy was having trouble with.

"One day, he was on his way to a client he'd had for years, and he got lost. He never kept the appointment—just disappeared for the whole day. When he finally came home that night, he couldn't remember where he'd been. And, of course, his boss had been on the telephone with me all day, trying to locate him.

"After that, they had to let him go. Actually it was very nice the way they handled it—getting him to retire and giving him a nice present and his pension and everything.

"But Sammy can't remember that he doesn't work anymore. He gets up every morning, early, and he puts his clothes on and starts to go out the door. And I tell him, 'Sammy, you don't have to go to work today.' But in five minutes he's forgotten. He starts with me: 'When do I go to work?' 'Am I going to work today?' 'Isn't it time to go to work?' Finally I got so frustrated with him—I mean, if I'd said it once, I've said it hundreds of times: 'You're retired, you don't have to go in anymore'—that I shoved him away from the door as he was trying to leave. And he turned around and he pushed me, straight across the room! Look at me, I'm black and blue!"

Unfortunately, in situations such as that of Sammy and his sister, her anger at him triggered an angry response from him. To keep her angry feelings from causing further trouble, she must find some constructive way to deal with her frustration.

These are the comments of some caregivers who have learned how they can best discharge some of their tension.

"I go out into the garage, and I get a hammer and a piece of wood and whang the daylights out of it."

"I bought a great big pillow and I keep it in my room, where my husband doesn't go. When he really gets to me, I go and punch it for a while."

If possible, try to get away for a little while; take a walk, if you can leave the patient alone, or telephone a friend. Better yet, ask the friend to stop over and give you a chance to get out for a few minutes, or just go next door to the neighbors. Some caregivers have found it helpful to scrub floors, or to polish furniture vigorously, or, when possible, to spend an hour in an active physical sport. Running, hitting tennis balls, or riding a bicycle for several miles are other ways that help to discharge the tension that is stored when we are angry.

Once the anger has dissipated, we are then in a better frame of mind to try to figure out why a particular behavior, or what set of circumstances, caused us to fly off the handle.

It helps to understand our feelings so that we can accept them and control the way we express them. Anger can be a constructive force, mobilizing us to protect ourselves and to assert ourselves when it is necessary and appropriate to do so. Yet anger is probably one of the most maligned of human emotions. When we are angry we are seen by others as immature, unhealthy, primitive, and a danger to ourselves and to society.

But to show our anger toward someone we love, in response to actions that he is no longer able to control, and for which he is therefore not accountable, is to use anger destructively. Ultimately, we may become self-destructive and then wind up hating ourselves for our behavior. We are also limiting our ability to help the person for whom we are caring. Anger replaces the lovingness we felt in the past. It makes the daily routines of feeding, bathing, dressing, and constant watchfulness even more frustrating and exhausting. To add misery upon misery, we also feel guilty because our lack of control led to further discord.

Moreover, the guilt over our angry outburst tends to persist long after we've made amends for our behavior, as happened with Mr. Kucera when he fought with his brother. Because we feel so guilty, we become less able to give ourselves "time off," and more and more trapped into caring for this totally dependent person, to the point of our own exhaustion. Thus guilt, sooner or later, contributes to our feeling more frustrated. And then, once again, we burn with anger.

To interrupt that vicious circle of anger/blowup/guilt/more anger, it helps to look at the circumstances that led us to feel angry in the first place. Understanding what was so infuriating about a certain behavior demystifies it and helps us recognize our wrathful feelings and manage them constructively in similar circumstances in the future.

Consider, for a moment, Ms. Bates's story of the morning when she pushed Sammy and he pushed her, when she got angry because he kept trying to go to work. A more helpful tactic might have been to soothe him affectionately and then divert his attention. For example, she might have said, "You would like to go to work today, but you don't have to. Come over here and look at these photographs with me," thus expressing empathy and then distracting him. Instead, on that occasion, her frustration boiled over into anger. Everyone experiences angry feelings from time to time. For Sammy's sister, understanding her disappointment and frustration because Sammy can no longer meet her own needs will help her to handle herself and Sammy more constructively.

To gain that understanding, she must look beyond the immediate moment and consider her deeper feelings. Here is a brother who has been a source of support and strength to her all her life. They grew up together, raised children in neighboring houses, and once again lived together in their adult years. In many ways their later life was like a mature marriage. He provided the income, he did household repairs, he was her major companion. Now, he can't work, he doesn't listen to her when she tells him the simplest thing, he can't handle tools or help around the house. She has been accustomed to depending on him for almost all of her needs for half a century, and now, suddenly, when she feels she needs him even more as she grows older, he is no longer there for her. She feels betrayed, disappointed, and fearful of being left alone when she can no longer care for him at home and must put him in a nursing home.

These feelings—the loneliness, the sense of betrayal and disappointment, the fear of loss—may underlie her overall anger at Sammy. The characteristic "straw that breaks the camel's back" and triggers a display of anger is her being thwarted or frustrated by Sammy's apparent disregard of what she tells him.

For the caregiver such as Ms. Bates, being aware of the true cause of her angry feelings and knowing how to cope with them will, one hopes, help her to understand herself. Then taking care of her memory-impaired brother will be less threatening and less frustrating.

Getting angry is not "bad" or reprehensible. It happens to every one of us when something in the behavior of our patient stimulates feelings of pain or fear that we haven't recognized or examined before. Sometimes it's not too easy to see why a certain act has upset us so. However, when the meaning of that act is understood in relation to our feelings about ourselves, then we no longer need be angry. Especially, when, as in Ms. Bates's case, our own needs go unmet and we feel frustrated, it becomes increasingly important for us to figure out why we are impatient or angry at the present moment. Once the source of the anger has been identified, remaining calm is easier, and thus it becomes easier to reassure an agitated relative.

Adults who, as children, were never allowed to express anger are often at a loss as to how to show it. There are acceptable ways to show anger, which is a normal, legitimate emotion. It is possible to express anger verbally, without necessarily destroying a relationship with another person, and without having to lose control of yourself.

Sharing feelings and experiences with a confidant or with a group can prevent you from experiencing an enormous sense of isolation if you "lose your cool" and resort to abusive behavior. Knowing that other people in the group have reacted in similar ways may alleviate some of the pain of guilt that caregivers experience after a blowup.

In a group therapy situation, both the psychotherapist and the other group members may be able to suggest healthier ways to handle problems as they arise.

An understanding and empathic attitude from the therapist and the group members diminishes some of the caregiver's tensions. Tension or anxiety emanates from fears of what might happen to the relative. A fear that can be paralyzing is that what is happening to the family member could happen to the caregiver as well. Such fears and resulting pressures often increase the caregiver's impatience and anger.

If we understand anger as a choice we make, a way in which we decide to express our frustration, rather than as something that just happens to us, we may be able to do something about our anger. Our emotions are, in essence, the physiological expression of our thoughts. Rather than letting our angry feelings turn into depression and immobilize us, we can learn how to manage and use anger in the interest of our survival.

CHAPTER 7

Depression: Longing for What Is Lost

MR. NATHANIEL GOULD: "My wife Molly and I met in music school, nearly fifty years ago. Neither of us ever became professional musicians, but we have always enjoyed going to concerts two or three times a week.

"But the last few concerts we attended were very distressing because Molly got impatient and restless and couldn't sit still. She said she felt sick, so we had to leave during the performance. I disliked disturbing the other people at the concert.

"Last Sunday we had tickets for an opera. My sister was visiting, so I asked her if she would care to go, but she wasn't particularly interested. Then I asked her if she would mind if I left Molly with her while I went by myself, and she agreed. So I went to the opera and relaxed and enjoyed it because I didn't have to worry about Molly becoming restless. At the same time, I won't have that freedom too often, so I think I will have to give up our subscriptions next season. I'll miss the concerts, but I already miss the fact that I can't share them with Molly. I've lost my companion."

MS. HELENA DORFMAN: "My father was in wonderful shape until he was 83. Even after he retired from his firm, he kept working. He and his good friend Todd, who had also been in the firm, formed a consulting business to work with other companies in the steel alloy industry. They shared an office until the day Todd died. Dad began to decline right after that, and I've always wondered if it was the grief that caused him to get sick.

"He's still at home with my mother, but I live a thousand miles away. When I took the children to visit Mom and Dad last month, he didn't recognize me. He didn't recognize any of us. We spent a week there, and it was so sad! He didn't speak to any of us, not once, until we were getting ready to leave. Then, out of nowhere, he said to my two youngest sons, 'Remember, I'm still the same old Grandpa!' I cried all the way to the airplane."

Ms. Merilee Tyler: "I've just learned from the doctor that my mother has something called Alzheimer's disease. This afternoon I went to the library and read all the articles that I could find on it. Right now she forgets where she puts things, and when she went to the store last week she got lost and wandered around town for half the day. But the articles all say that she will forget more and more and become increasingly incapable of caring for herself. It's so depressing to think about that. Must it really happen?"

Mr. Gould has lost his companion of fifty years, Ms. Dorfman, her loving father, Ms. Tyler will eventually lose her mother, as her mother loses her memory. They are all experiencing losses, which precipitate feelings of depression.

What Is Depression?

From time to time, everyone feels blue, unhappy, discouraged, worried, listless, nervous, irritable, filled with anguish, self-disgust, and intense guilt. These emotional states are painful. You feel miserable when these painful feelings return day after day and the sadness feels like a "heavy heart." If you feel weary, agitated, hopeless, or unnerved by small obstacles, if your appetite has disappeared and your sleep is disturbed, you are probably experiencing some form of depression. Depression is both a physical and emotional experience. It means that you have been unable to adapt to the stresses of life.

The body generally shows the strain first, developing any number of physical complaints as depression reduces your efficiency and disturbs your appetite and your sleep. Subsequently, the intellectual and emotional systems weaken, affecting your abilities to think, work, or remember.

Common physical symptoms of which depressed people frequently complain include the following:

- Headache
- Dizziness, fainting
- Blurred vision
- Rapid heartbeat
- Loss of body control (dropping things)
- Trouble breathing (tightness across the chest)
- A burning sensation at the top and back of the head
- Constipation or diarrhea
- Pressure in the bladder
- Colicky pains in the bladder
- Heartburn or nausea
- Stomach spasms
- Pains in the chest (mistaken for heart attack)
- Aches and cramps in the legs and back
- Sweating
- Itching or tingling sensations in the skin
- Weakness in body/shakiness

These physical symptoms are the body's signals of distress. A depressed person is alerted by his physical warning system when he psychologically denies his emotional reactions and feelings. Thus depression can be understood as a sign that we feel we have lost ourselves. That feeling is extremely painful. A person who is depressed sees himself as a failure. His self-esteem is very fragile because he lacks confidence in his own thoughts, ideas, and feelings. He usually seeks perfection in himself, so he is very critical of his own performance. The same is true about how he sees other people. When he fails to live up to his own high standards or when others disappoint him, his oversensitivity makes him feel shameful and very guilty.

The depressed person has an enormous fear of losing the love of people upon whom he is dependent for affection and caring. Therefore he conforms to the needs and wishes of these people even if they conflict with his own. Such conformity requires that his own interests be suppressed or denied. The price of such dependency is resentment and anger. Thus the depressed person is, in reality, a very angry person; he is angry at himself.

Unaware of his anger which he has repressed, or unable to acknowledge his angry feelings, instead he turns the anger inward. It becomes aggression against himself. But actually the angry feelings cover up a deep sense of disappointment in himself. And, thus, he becomes sad, or depressed.

As children, depressed adults were probably not free to express discontent or disappointment. Unrelieved frustration soon turns to anger and rage. But, unable to express either of these painful emotions for fear of losing mother's love, the child becomes depressed, looking mournful and feeling sad.

Healthy emotions are useful to us. For example, when there is a threat to our security or survival, the emotion of anxiety may mobilize us to take constructive action. Anxious about failing a driving test, we study the driver's manual and take more lessons until we improve our driving skills and can pass the test. Anger at life's injustices may motivate us to become better citizens by championing what we feel are "good causes" and help us to deal more fairly with our children.

However, when we cannot deal with a potentially overwhelming situation, we may become flooded by our fears, anxieties, and anger. Then we may respond to the threat of illness (our own depression or the continuing decline of our memory-impaired relative) with restlessness and a panic reaction. We may be filled with dread, always anticipating the worst. Fear of being left alone, fear of failure, rage at being ill, irritation, sarcasm, and blaming others for one's own distress are all manifestations of the depression that hides beneath such erratic behaviors. Real sadness, pain, and self-deprecation are the underlying feelings of the person who is depressed.

A depressed person's thoughts sometimes become distorted. He fears and often says he's afraid of "going crazy." Often the fear is that he will pass along his depression to other members of the family. There is no clear evidence that depression is inherited. However, children who are brought up in households where either parent was chronically depressed may be more susceptible to depression because they have learned behavior patterns of the depressed person (learned helplessness).

Not all of us let our depressed feelings show. Thus it is sometimes a shock to us to hear that someone who has never seemed particularly sad, hopeless, or depressed has tried to commit suicide. Often, people who have never appeared to be depressed have successfully hidden their depressed feelings from themselves as well as from others until the moment when those feelings of sadness and helplessness overwhelm them.

Some depressions are mildly distressing and can be overcome rather quickly. People with moderate, acute, or recurrent severe depression can benefit from the assistance of psychotherapists and psychoanalysts. In cases of very severe depression, the person may, at the same time, benefit from seeing a psychiatrist or a physician who can prescribe an antidepressant medication. Such drugs give the depressed person immediate relief but should be used for brief periods of time only. They are most useful in conjunction with psychotherapy and should not be used as the only method of treating the depressed person.

An acute depression may come on quickly, last a week or a few months, and then clear up. Recurrent depressions appear at irregular intervals and last indefinitely, sometimes years. Some depressions slow a person down; others, which are agitated states of depression, keep one in a state of general nervous excitement.

Why Older People Get Depressed

With increased longevity, older people lack role models that are appropriate. As we grow older, we find ourselves encountering many difficulties for which we are ill prepared. Retirement, the "empty nest," changes in society, the death of friends or parents, the need to relocate to a new environment, and chronic illness all play a part in the depression that may occur with aging. Physical changes that affect and reduce the circulation of blood to the brain may also lead to depression.

The older person usually experiences depression as a sense of loss. Feeling depressed or sad as a reaction to loss is both a normal and universal phenomenon. Since all people face losses from time to time, everyone may experience some depression in his lifetime. There are many occasions when we expect to feel depressed; for example, when someone close dies, at the end of a love affair, when a business fails, or after losing a job or an expected prize or award.

Depression tends to be less noticeable in the older person than it is in the young. If you are caring for a person with Alzheimer's disease and notice such symptoms or behaviors in yourself, you may become frightened and think you also have the disease or are depressed. But remember, depression touches many adult lives at some time. Depression is a treatable illness, and the symptoms are reversible. If there are times when *you* feel apathetic, irritable, or confused, try to understand what is causing these feelings. Assuming that apathy, mental confusion, and irritability either are expected because we are aging or are the unalterable signs of organic disease sentences thousands of people unnecessarily to painful dependency and impaired functioning.

There are many losses caused by external circumstances that can precipitate a depression. Some are quite obvious, but others are less so. For an older person in particular, the most frequently experienced disappointments are in the reality he previously had been able to count on. He could make order out of chaos and believe in the idea of the goodness of all people.

The values of mutual cooperation are being eroded by the younger generation's self-absorbed attitude, which reflects the changing times in our culture. Awareness of the differences in philosophical ideals and social attitudes contributes to the older person's feelings of emptiness. It leads to the loss of a reliable internal sense of the self. As former ideals and attitudes are challenged by society, the older person's self-esteem diminishes. As a result, he may react with enormous rage. Rage pushes other people away and reduces the number of meaningful relationships that can be enjoyed with the people who are important in our lives.

Other losses that impair the older person's self-esteem and contribute to a devalued self-image and decreased self-confidence are due to the aging process. The loss of one's talent, physical attractiveness, memory, or a bodily function; diminished eyesight or hearing; reduced precision in hand-and-finger skills through arthritis; for men, impotence, or any curb on the ability to satisfy his sexual needs; confinement to bed during a chronic illness and the resulting awareness of loss of mobility and freedom; the inability to tolerate the aging process itself; and the idea of the inevitability of death—any and all such losses may lead to depression. When the losses and restrictions are temporary, and the underlying conditions can be treated and improved, when skills and health are restored, then the depression may lift as well.

Fears of overdoing it and harming oneself physically are often restraints that cause depression in older people. Fear of having a heart attack or a stroke may lead to decreased activity on the part of the older person.

> Ms. Agatha Conover: "My Dad always loved gardening. His parents had been florists, and his house never looked right to him unless it was surrounded by bedding plants which were appropriate to the season. Two years ago he had a heart attack, and although the doctor says he's fully recovered, he still worries about it. He fears that if he pushes the wheelbarrow around, full of plants and soil, especially in the hot summer sun, he might have another attack. So he has stopped planting his garden with seasonal flowers. His feeling of apprehension about his health has deprived him unnecessarily of one of his greatest pleasures—seeing his house and yard in all its summer glory."

Cautious behavior on the part of spouses and other relatives can further inhibit the activities of the elderly person. The reduction of freedom and independence may make the elderly person feel depressed, and as his depression increases, he may view more and more aspects of the outside world as threatening or frightening.

A retired architect was in the habit of visiting a nearby museum every week. The museum entrance was at the head of a long flight of steep steps.

Although he had never had any trouble getting to the top of the steps, after he had a brief bout with pneumonia his children and grandchildren began to insist that the long flight of stairs would be too much for him. They told him that if he insisted on going to the museum, he should at least rest on his way up the steps. On his next visit he took the steps more slowly, resting every dozen or so. He felt conspicuous and feeble and embarrassed as he leaned on the bannister. Once inside the museum, he found that he couldn't enjoy the paintings he had come to see because he was worried about going home.

As he dutifully rested on his way down the steps, he noticed several young people nearby who seemed to be studying him closely. He became conscious of his expensive watch, the money in his wallet, and his visible weakness. He had never carried a cane in his life, but he wished he had one for possible defense.

Thereafter, his visits to the museum became fewer. He became more and more bored and unhappy, but at the same time less and less willing to venture out on his own. Whenever he did go out, he felt threatened and apprehensive.

Sex, Intimacy, and Depression

Whether your loss is the usefulness of a part of your body, another person, a keepsake, a symbol of independence such as your own home, or a familiar role, you have lost something that is an important contribution to your self-definition, to your happiness and satisfaction. Losing someone or something of significance plays a role in depression. In addition to all the above, caregivers are faced with the almost overwhelming, undeniable loss of the memory and companionship of the memory-impaired person.

As we grow older, many things happen to us that seem to threaten our independence, our self-esteem, and our continued ability to function.

Physical infirmities reduce our skill and competence with daily tasks. The death or impairment of a beloved spouse makes us question whether we can continue to live alone. Friends move farther away, so we can't call on them as readily as companionship and emotional support. The very perception that such events are threatening to us can lead to depression. That depression, in turn, can cause a person who suffers from it to feel more threatened by events.

There are situations in which society itself tries to limit our capabilities or their expression. For example, there is an attitude prevailing in our culture that the elderly are sexless, or asexual, people. Or, if they are not sexless, then they must be the stereotypical "dirty old man" or "dirty old lady." These cruel perceptions of loving, mature sexuality may cause older people to restrict their sexual activity. The fear of criticism or the threat of ridicule may influence them to feel less free to express their sexual needs.

However, when we consider the many sources of depression in older people, it is worth noting that the relationship between sex and depression in the elderly is an inverse one. The more interest an older person has in sex and the more opportunity he has to participate as a sexual being, the less depressed he is. Orgasm has the power to confirm and to recreate our own reality. Thus enhanced sexual interest and activity can be an antidote to depression.

On the other hand, any disappointment where your wishes are not granted after you have anticipated great satisfaction is a loss that can lead to depression. Seduction by a spouse or friend that does not lead to a fulfilling sexual experience or an opportunity for satisfaction is such a loss. Madeleine Jarrett's loss of her husband's ability to respond to her as an adult disappoints all her hopes for a companionate old age.

"I've become a mother to my husband instead of a wife. I find it's difficult to make this change in role at this point in my life. In the attempt, I feel I'm not my usual self. I seem to have other thoughts that are taking over. They're sad and depressing, and I don't like the feeling.

"I feel very sorry for myself because I can't become what my husband needs me to be. I don't have the commitment, as you must, for example, for a sick child, that doesn't stop, no matter how old or young or sick that child may be. I don't have the strength any more to be a 'mother' in that way, and certainly not to my husband."

We remain strongly attached to our loved ones whom we have virtually lost even after we have admitted that the loss is irretrievable. As a caregiver to someone with Alzheimer's disease, even though you know intellectually that your relative is "lost to you forever," you may find yourself unable to form other liaisons because you still feel all the emotional ties and responsibilities that bind you to your patient.

If you are taking care of an impaired husband or wife, and another person happens to show an emotional or sexual interest in you, you may well be unwilling or unable to abandon your feelings of love and your investment of energy in your spouse. Hence, the epithet "married widows and widowers" that some caregiving spouses have attached to themselves. They still feel bound to their spouses, even though that spouse may be merely vegetating, or existing physically without any memory of an emotional attachment.

> MRS. ADELE MICKELJON: "He doesn't care. He doesn't care about anyone or anything now. He used to be crazy about the grandchildren. He's forgotten them. It used to be if they called up and said, 'Grandpa, I want a toy, or a train,'—or anything—he would drop whatever he was doing and go buy it for them. Now, when he sees them—nothing.
>
> "I ask him, 'Do you know who this is? It's your grandson.'
> " 'Oh.'
>
> "Half the time he doesn't recognize me. When we're walking together, sometimes he'll stop and say, 'I'm waiting for my wife. Where is my wife? What have you done with her?' That gives me a horrible feeling."

As Mr. Mickeljon becomes less and less the person he once was, Mrs. Mickeljon finds herself grieving for the person she married, for the person who gave comfort, and pride, and companionship. Even though that person is still physically alive, the fabric of the relationship, which depends so much on remembrance of the past, has for the most part vanished.

Intimacy between a husband and wife may also be lost if your spouse is afflicted with Alzheimer's disease or another form of memory impairment. People who are memory-impaired still engage in sexual activity with their spouses when their spouses permit them to do so. But while the sexual act may be a source of satisfaction to the patient, the caregiver may feel repulsed. Alzheimer's patients often seem to have fewer cultural and social inhibitions than most of their unafflicted peers. The healthy caregiving spouse, however, frequently finds it difficult to participate sexually when the emotional aspects of the relationship are missing. Many women complain that they are being used as sexual objects by their afflicted spouses, while getting no sexual satisfaction themselves. Other women feel that their spouse has so few pleasures that they participate sexually merely to give comfort to their partner.

> MRS. ARDIS CARROLL: "My husband was a wonderful, tender, thoughtful, and considerate lover. But since he became ill, for two years I've had absolutely no physical or emotional satisfaction. I don't get anything from the sexual experience. We do it and get it over with quickly, and that's that. Afterwards, I feel degraded. It's as if we were rutting in the backyard."

Some husbands and wives reject the sexual overtures of a memory-impaired spouse because the total relationship is affected by the illness. Unable to communicate with their spouses, they no longer feel comfortable making love. Also, a caregiver who is totally involved in attending to an Alzheimer's patient's daily needs may be too tired or too depressed to be interested in sex.

Before the issue of too much, too little, or no sex at all looms large in your married life, if you are caring for a memory-impaired person, you would be well advised to seek professional sexual counseling.

While caregivers often turn to physicians for information about how to react to the confused person's sexual overtures, physicians, unfortunately, are rarely equipped with the knowledge they need to provide

85

such counseling. Many physicians, furthermore, are extremely reluctant to explore this intimate aspect of their patients' lives.

Reputable psychotherapists and sex therapists, however, are prepared to discuss the vicissitudes of this delicate subject. If they have had experience working with the elderly and are knowledgeable about Alzheimer's disease and similar disorders and the effects of such handicaps on sexual behavior, they will be able to discuss the issues sensitively and offer some guidance. The spouse who is sexually starved but deprived of a willing companion might benefit from instruction in autoeroticism or masturbation techniques that provide some sexual pleasure and a decrease in sexual tensions. The spouse who wishes to develop new or additional bonds of affection or to make other sexual contacts may need to discuss feelings of guilt about "such a terribly selfish desire when my poor wife is so ill." To yearn for and seek warmth, caring, affection, and sexual satisfaction is not wrong or despicable. It is merely an acknowledgment that, despite the burdens weighing heavily on us, we are still human and crave the most human of emotions: to be wanted, cared for, loved, to feel and express physical passion.

Caregivers also experience feelings of loneliness and social isolation as they discover themselves alone with their burdens. They withdraw from friends and other relationships; other people, in turn, withdraw from them.

MR. MEL HART: "There are days when I hate to come home from work. My wife, Georgina, is home all the time. There's never a telephone call or a visit from anyone. It's a lonesome existence. I've quit asking her friends to call her, but when they all come to her funeral they'll say what a wonderful woman she was. It hurts me, even though I know that our friends can't stand to see what's happened to Georgina, and so they stay away."

GERRY VOIGHT: "My father's family won't come to visit. They say things like, 'My brother is not the same person that he was.' Even his sister Carol, who lives only five minutes away. . . . Dad supported her when she was younger and had some money problems, but now?

"I hear my mother talking on the telephone with Aunt Carol: 'You're just five minutes away. You walk by the house every day on your way home from the bus. Can't you just stop off for a few minutes? You don't have to make it a big deal, or even talk to me if you don't want to. But please, just stop by and say hello to your brother, then go!' She never does."

Many caregivers find that other family members withdraw from them because they are appalled by the impaired person and do not like to witness his sometimes bizarre behavior. On the other hand, some caregivers tend to withdraw from friends who seem to them not to understand their predicament or their relative's situation.

Ms. HARRIET SAUNDERS: "I have lost my friends. I didn't want to see that pitying look on their faces, as they asked, 'Gee, what happened to that wonderful man . . . ?'

"Today, whatever friends I have are only those friends who will talk to Johnny just like they used to. Even though he doesn't answer them, maybe they feel that he understands; they don't look down on him. I won't have them talk to him as if he were an imbecile. There are a few people I enjoy having around, but all the others—I've given up their society."

Stress Reactions in Caregivers

Each day, every week, month, and year that your relative remains ill or deteriorates further, you mourn the loss of that person. At some point during the course of a relative's illness, many caregivers begin to feel useless and helpless. Subsequently they may experience apathy, listlessness, nervousness, irritability, decreased physical vitality and mental energy, and an overall decrease in stamina. Matilda Howard's day may sound familiar.

"My mother and I went to the new Smithsonian exhibit yesterday. She was perfect! She was lively, she commented on the exhibit. We had no disagreements at all. But as soon as we got back to her apartment, she began to ask me the same questions she asked me this morning, which were the same questions I answered for her yesterday.

"I get so frustrated. I know I should have patience, but this has been going on for over a year. If anything, it's getting worse. I don't know how much longer I can cope before I crack up!

"There were some clean towels in the clothes dryer. First she folded them—the wrong way—then, instead of putting them away, she pulled everything else out of the linen closet.

"'Please!' I said. 'Let's just have one day—just one—when I can have a rest!' I had reorganized that closet for her the day before yesterday!

"Meanwhile, I have nothing but turmoil in my own house. I used to be so neat, and so did she! My own linen closet is in disarray. I had promised myself I would organize it after I did hers, but when I got home I didn't have the patience. I just wasn't in the mood. I was so tired. So it's still a mess.

"I used to feel that I was so strong I could do almost anything. Now I neglect my own concerns. I'm so depressed that I can't think straight. I can't concentrate on anything.

"I can't accept my mother as she is, I just cannot! I never thought that she might not always be as competent and independent as she has always been. My friends have said to me, 'She's in wonderful shape, in perfect health at 78. You don't know how good you have it.' I believed them. Now she's not what she was for me.

"I miss her being able to be a mother to me, but I also miss the communication. I reproach myself for telling her something in a way that it doesn't penetrate.

"When she talks to me sometimes she hesitates, then thinks a while, and then she tells me her thoughts. I always wait for her. But when I talk to her, if I hesitate for just a moment, she's right on top of me, finishing my sentence. She fills in what I want to say. I get very annoyed, and accuse her of not listening to me. She doesn't understand. She just says, 'But it takes you so long!' She thinks she's helping me. It's been that way since I was a child.

"I feel sad because I'm so critical of her now, and I never used to be. There was a time when she could do no wrong. And if she did do something to annoy me, I would never admit it.

"She can remember intellectual things, like the theme of the Smithsonian show, or current events, or cultural happenings. It's the day-to-day things around the apartment that confuse her.

"It's reaching a point where I just can't continue going through this day after day. I don't do anything that's fun any more. I don't allow myself to. I always enjoyed it better when Mother participated, even though she often irritated me. She has been very generous and good to me, and I feel that she deserves to be catered to. But I can't do it any more. I've failed. I'm not a patient daughter.

"I'm very depressed about it. I tell her that. She says, 'Why are you angry with me?' and I answer, 'Because it hurts me to see you when you act or are, helpless.'

"But the real problem is my own helplessness. I can't help her!"

Unfortunately, when we care for a memory-impaired person, we may exceed our own physical and emotional capacities. Driven by feelings of love, devotion, or duty, we may forget about our own needs. When we surrender our own personal interests, ignore all other obligations (to other family members, children or spouse, friends or employer), and neglect getting enough sleep and good food, we impinge on our own time for rest and relaxation. Then we put ourselves in situations of chronic stress that can propel us right into a depression. At the same time, identification with the confused patient (a "There but for the grace of God go I" attitude) may lead us to "experience" the patient's suffering as if it were our own. This additional stress can lead to a total exhaustion of our inner resources.

Ms. Howard could accept neither her mother's illness nor her own feelings about the illness. She depleted her energies in her efforts to help her mother and wound up feeling helpless and depressed herself.

Most of the depressions that caregivers experience are "reactive"— that is, they are precipitated by the illness of the loved one. As the mental condition of the Alzheimer's patient continues to deteriorate, the changes in the patient make it vividly apparent to the caregiver both that the illness will affect his total future and well-being and that his relative is lost to him. The impact of being deprived of that formerly loving, nurturing, and responsive parent, spouse, in-law, or friend changes the caregiver's basic way of life. When caregivers react to their painful frustration with grief, they may begin prematurely to mourn the loss of the beloved.

The sense of loss is the essence of the reactive depression. The loss is so great that the caregiver may respond with inconsolable mourning or grief. When a husband and wife have been extremely dependent on one another, the sense of loss experienced by the healthy spouse may increase his depression. If the relationship was unequal, and the dominant partner becomes ill, the dependent spouse, who must now become the caregiver, may not be able to handle the new responsibilities and, as a result, can become depressed.

Being depressed is such a painful experience that the wish for relief becomes foremost in the mind of the caregiver. As Ms. Howard said: "Please! Let's just have one day—just one!—when I can have a rest!" Many of us feel like that—completely overwhelmed by the misery of the day-and-night vigils and the despairing feelings over someone we love.

Lifting the Depression

It is only by being able to tolerate the feeling of sorrow and the sense of loss that we may be able to express the depression. Thinking about today and taking each day as it comes may reduce the sense of loss. Deriving satisfaction from small, immediate pleasures can mitigate against a dim, long-term view of the realistic limitations of our lives.

Sharing feelings of loss with close friends or relatives can be helpful. In addition, sharing your experiences and emotions with other caregivers in a psychotherapy group can help you to cope with the depression that arises in the daily care of a patient.

Sometimes relatives turn away from a depressed person because he seems to make inordinate demands upon them, tries to manipulate them, and rarely smiles or gives any sign of gratitude for their attention to him. Negative interactions contribute to hostility and tension between the depressed person and other family members. When relatives or friends feel empathy for the depressed person and wish to be helpful, they may hesitate to speak for fear of saying the wrong thing. Unfortunately, they may not realize how very helpful it is to hear expressions of empathy verbalized.

Well-meaning friends who don't understand your plight may say the wrong thing. Ignore them. Don't berate yourself for feeling sad and lonely just because someone else tells you to pull yourself together or quit feeling sorry for yourself.

HELPING YOURSELF OUT OF A MILD DEPRESSION

The inability to take action is a characteristic of depression. The depressed person cannot think of anything he would enjoy doing. To alleviate mild depression we may be able to find things that satisfy us at least in our fantasy.

Imagine several things that will give you satisfaction, such as food, hobbies, entertainment, sex, travel, work, social interactions. Look for the most minute things that may give the smallest feeling of pleasure or larger things like winning a prize or a loving relationship that makes you feel good.

Then choose one of the acts that is especially pleasurable and imagine yourself doing it—for example, dining out in a nice restaurant. Try to experience the good feelings you imagine.

Do this exercise daily until you relieve your depression to the degree that you may repeat your fantasy in real life (actually dine out).

Now that you are starting to control your depression, try to increase your daily activities so that you can eventually find new sources of pleasure. List those events that you enjoyed very much at one time. These activities may range from telephone visiting to shopping trips with friends, dining out, or going for a walk. Give yourself a specific time

91

and date that you'll perform the activity. Write yourself a note about it and make a contract with yourself. Start by doing one action each week—you must do it! Pay attention to any pleasurable feeling you may get from the activity. It will reawaken your awareness of pleasant feelings. In your depressed state, you have learned to ignore these feelings just as you've learned to be helpless. The result of this experience is that you'll become more action-oriented and learn to take responsibility for putting pleasure into your life.

If Your Depression Gets Worse

You may not be able to keep from crying some of the time if your depression increases. Crying does relieve some of the ache, but it is also exhausting and can sap your energy and reduce your stamina.

At times you may become tremendously anxious about the smallest things. It may be frightening to be alone. When people are sad, lonely, and depressed, they may become preoccupied with thoughts of their own death. It is important to remember that during a depression the nervous system does not function correctly, and thoughts tend to be rigid. These thoughts can become obsessional and make us fearful that we may harm ourselves. Even though you don't really want to die, you may have a premonition about your own death.

The risk of suicide is great in all depressed people, especially those with severe depression. You should not stay alone, although you may want to. Until a depressed person is well on his way to recovery, he may become self-destructive. A calm statement such as "I could walk into the ocean until my hat floats" may be more indicative of a potential suicide threat than a wailing and hysterical scream of "God take me out of my misery." The rising tension and loss of hope is what precipitates most suicide attempts. All suicide threats and attempts should be taken seriously by those who hear them.

Because of the cyclical nature of depression, you will feel better in time. However, it is advisable not to wait, but to seek treatment immediately. You can find support, encouragement, and understanding without waiting for eventual relief. Although friends and relatives can help by being supportive and sympathetic, they are rarely able to be objective, an important characteristic of an experienced psychotherapist. The psychotherapist can offer support, encouragement, and vitalizing assurance. A competent psychotherapist knows what depression is all about and will help to sustain you in your despair. Knowing that the therapist is available to you when necessary and that the therapist is interested in your welfare will help you feel comforted. Anxiety will recede as you recognize that you are not struggling alone.

The depressed person who feels guilty and locks all his guilts away needs a place to release these powerful feelings and get them out of his system. This is the release, or catharsis, that is spoken about in psychotherapy. It is similar to a confession or unburdening, which lessens the weight of emotional burdens. It may be that you are overly conscientious. This is often true of people who are caregivers to patients with Alzheimer's disease. Overzealousness may arise from inner feelings of guilt (or an overly strict conscience) about past errors, unkindness, or desertions. Feelings of insecurity or deprivation that culminate in repressed anger can also make one feel guilty. The caregiver who, because of guilt, sacrifices himself, in turn overprotects his patient and creates unnecessary dependency in the patient.

A proper diagnosis is essential, followed by positive treatment. The psychotherapist will explain to you why you feel sluggish, have no appetite, can't sleep, are worried, or seem to have constant aches and pains. After taking your history, the therapist may call upon members of your family to see what aggravations there are in your whole environment. You will have an opportunity to talk about your distressing thoughts and feelings that interfere with everyday living. The therapist will encourage you to expect less of yourself and help you find ways to become more relaxed and less driven in your view of life.

Your therapist can be helpful in other ways: by advising family members and friends to give you more time for relaxation and to reduce family tensions; by helping you to put these unhappy months in the larger perspective of your life, by reminding you that you have handled other problems successfully; by suggesting a program of physical activity to release your tensions and raise your spirits; and by helping you to insightful self-understanding. Through these insights and suggestions you will feel better about yourself and your life. Psychotherapy is a process of exploration, support, and reeducation. Thus it requires time, effort, and patience in order for the process to be effective and for the depressed person to recover.

CHAPTER 8

Guilt: A Nagging Pain

Since the days of our early childhood, we carry within us a model of goodness and a fear of disapproval from our parents. We incorporate parental values, which ultimately become the primary motivation for socially acceptable behavior.

Thus, the purpose of conscience is to make the individual responsible to the group. (The group may be one's family, community, or country.) Through identification with the group, we develop a social conscience. Conscience helps us to feel good about ourselves when we are in harmony with the original standards and values of our parents (now translated as society's values). But, when we err or behave selfishly and not in the interest of others, we may be faced with a self-inflicted punishment. The punishment is a nagging pain that can become a constant companion. That nagging pain is a feeling of guilt. Guilt tells us we do not approve of our own behavior.

MR. EVANS: "Although I was always more outgoing than my wife, the differences between us seem to have become more marked since she became ill. We got invited to go for a daytrip to the Poconos with the local AARP group, but my wife doesn't want to go anywhere. She would rather just be left home alone. So I don't think I'll be able to go.

"I leave her alone for a few hours a day, but to be away from early morning until late at night would make me feel real guilty. Maybe I shouldn't feel guilty. I've had weekends with 'the guys' all my life, so that doesn't bother me. But in this situation, I feel I'm taking advantage of her. Maybe she'll need something.

"It's hard to sort out all my feelings. If she were well, I'd insist that she go to the Poconos with me. Or, if she were well, and she didn't want to go, I'd still go, and it would be all right.

"But, considering her condition, I feel I should sacrifice for her. I feel guilty for leaving her alone and going away and enjoying the day when I know she can't."

Mr. Evans has been "well socialized"—that is, he behaves in socially accepted ways. He is not able to enjoy himself when his wife is ill because of his conscience.

How do we make sense out of things that happen to us that are beyond our control, such as illness and death of loved ones? Family members often blame themselves or each other, or the sick or dying person, in just such an attempt to understand the unknown.

The two Mr. Broders, father and son, thoughtfully tried to produce an explanation. Both intelligent businessmen, they were at a loss to explain why the elder Mr. Broder's wife had developed Alzheimer's disease.

FATHER: "She was healthy, she seemed happy at home preparing meals for us, doing the laundry, baking strudel, playing with her two grandchildren. Did we do something wrong? Maybe if we had insisted that she go out more, have more friends, read more, join the Ladies' Auxiliary. . . . "

SON: "But she was a loner; she liked her own company and she didn't have time for all these other things. She said that she wasn't interested, that her family was her greatest joy and fulfillment."

FATHER: "Maybe it wasn't enough. Oh, God, why did you make such misery fall on such a sweet woman, and on me? She hardly knows me anymore. She's not the same wonderful Rowena any more. What have I done? Maybe I deserve it."

Mr. Broder is conscience-stricken.

Is the Broder family really guilty. Would it have made a difference if Mrs. Broder had read more, talked more, been more involved in the outside environment? It is highly improbable, since Alzheimer's disease does not respect the class, education, or activities of its victims. All family members can be sources of emotional stress for each other. Sometimes they do interfere with each other's desires to develop various skills or interests, but certainly they have no influence over the development of a chronic illness.

Conscious or Unconscious Guilt

Sometimes we experience guilt over things we do knowingly, and of which we have conscious awareness. The child who steals cookies from the cookie jar knows that it's wrong to do so because he's been told so, many times. However, the child may reason that the punishment (a soft spanking) is worth the crime (taking the cookies). The child has made a conscious decision to do something wrong, feels guilty about it, and risks the inevitable punishment. In this sense the child recognizes his guilt (conscious guilt) and accepts the responsibility for his own action. Within the limits of the child's awareness, such an act shows emotional maturity.

Unconscious guilt is buried and comes to the surface in what seem like strange ways, as through our dreams. For example, on the way to pay a visit to her chronically ill mother, Carolyn Grosvenor detoured from the highway onto a road that led to the Botanical Garden. It was a hot sunny day in spring, and she wanted to buy some house plants for herself and perhaps one or two for her mother. As she pulled off the main road, she hit an oncoming car, dented her fender and got a flat tire. She spent two and a half hours waiting for her car to be fixed, and by that time had to return home to fix her husband's dinner. That night,

Carolyn had a dream that she was being chased and physically threatened by two men who looked like her husband and her father (both authority figures to Carolyn). In the dream her mother was helpless, fell out of bed, and died. Carolyn's dream suggests that she may have both wished for as well as feared her mother's death. Carolyn awakened from the dream feeling very guilty for resenting her mother and wishing she didn't have to devote so much time to taking care of her.

The unconscious guilt relates to Ms. Grosvenor's uncomfortable feelings about not really wanting to visit her mother that day. She feels irresponsible; yet the more guilt she feels about her mother, the harder it may be for her to act responsibly. By running away from the problem, she tries to dodge her guilty feelings. Usually it can't be done.

One way to make unconscious guilt come to the surface is through a session in psychotherapy. In one such session, as Evelyn Bronson tried to deal with the death of her father after a long bout with cancer, she tried to withhold her tears. Evelyn told about remodeling the house she had inherited from her father after his death a few months ago. In her hurry to get new flooring, tiling, a new couch, and doors, and to plan for her child's birthday party, she denied that she had a lot of feelings about these changes and the fact that her father would not be around for the happy occasion.

> "Plus I feel guilty because he asked me to get the kids something for Easter that they could remember him by. He knew he wouldn't be around for Easter. I never did it. I forgot . . . no, I just didn't have time to get anything for them."

No, that's not it, either. In reality, not getting the gifts was Evelyn's way of denying her father's impending death. Later she felt guilty because she didn't fulfill his wishes.

> MRS. GOLDBERGER: "We always dreamed about retiring and traveling together. My husband retired two years ago, and we immediately planned a trip to Switzerland, a place we'd always wanted to visit. It was the only trip we've been able to take because my father is ill. Even for that

vacation, we had to make special arrangements for someone to care for him. It's just too difficult to work it out. He doesn't like the aides who come in, he insults them and won't cooperate. So we've had to content ourselves with taking daytrips.

"We do spend a lot of time with Father. We don't desert him or put him in the hands of strangers. But whenever we go away, even for a little while, we feel guilty. We have one visiting nurse, the same woman whom he's known for four years, who comes in for the day when we go away. He likes her very much, but whenever we leave, he says, 'Don't worry about me. I'll be all right all alone.' That's not the way he used to be. He always used to say, 'Go and leave me alone. I don't need anybody.' Now he wants us around; he's become very dependent, and wants to have us there all the time. Our lives have changed so much because of this."

The Relationship between Parent and Child

Older parents often trigger guilt feelings in their middle-aged children through a word or merely with a gesture. As Mrs. Goldberger's father said, "Don't worry about me being here alone by myself." The implication is: "Worry about me and don't leave me."

"You run off and have fun, I'll be all right, I'd only be in the way," says one mother as she looks mournfully and sorrowfully away. This attitude has been expressed in the "Jewish mother" jokes the comedians use to illustrate how parents make children feel guilty for living independently from their parents. But it could be the Roman Catholic mother, the Irish mother, the black mother, or the Armenian father, or the Italian father, or any mother or father who is capable of the same guilt-evoking words or behavior.

What parent hasn't told his children, "Wait until you have children. See how you feel when they leave you out of their lives, when they tell you you're too old, or too slow, or too old-fashioned to understand!"

When children of any age wish for the death of their parents, it is usually because they are angry with their parents; then they feel too despicable to admit such feelings. However, when parents are old and infirm, or when a spouse is terminally ill or memory-impaired, a family member may wish for the death of that relative, either as a way of ending the suffering of that person or as a means of ending the suffering he feels, which saps his own emotional and physical strength.

In either case, whenever we wish for the death of a loved one, we are immediately burdened by feelings of guilt. We also feel guilty when we are unable to care for our relative in the same way we were cared for as youngsters:

> Ms. DODD: "My mother took care of me when I was small, so I feel that I'm supposed to do the same thing, because that's really what you're supposed to do—you're supposed to take care of your parents. I can't imagine that it is as intense between husband and wife, despite the marriage vows of 'till death do us part,' because you don't have the obligation from childhood. At least maybe the guilt in a marriage isn't quite as bad. Is that possible? It's so subjective. How do you measure guilt?"

A nursing home resident said it best when, after selling his home, he spent time in each of his ten children's homes and then decided to come to the nursing home: "One father can take care of ten children, but ten children can't take care of one father." And King Lear announced how much pain he suffered because of "thankless" children. Although they had divided his money, his power, and his kingdom, two of his three children did not want the burden of caring for this old and mentally failing man.

Parents often feel hurt by the ingratitude of their children, when parental nurturance and sacrifice go unrewarded. Although they say they expect little in return, parents do expect children to show some gratefulness. Children, on the other hand, get used to their parents' services and often do not regard them as more than their birthright and the parents' duty. Special occasions are usually the time children do express gratitude. Perhaps it is ironic that as children need fewer services from their parents, the parents' wish for some expression of gratitude increases. As parents approach the time when their nest will be empty, they fear they will no longer be needed; for some, the fear is they will no longer be loved. These fears may precipitate the demands for reassurances from their children. The reassurance is not only recognition for past services, but some acknowledgment that, should the parents need the child in the future, the child can be called upon. Without such assurances, the parents may feel hurt and in turn become angry with the child.

Faced with his anger at the children he loves, the needy parent may become confused, thinking that he does not love his children; then he feels very guilty. But instead of acknowledging the guilt or his angry feelings, he denies both.

We feel hurt when people we care about do not show concern for our feelings. If a supportive family member withdraws love and affection, it may be because we are expecting too much from that person.

There is a tendency to forget that people get responded to in kind— that is, in terms of how they behaved toward others. Very often older people living in nursing homes are devastated because their children don't come to visit them. Children have many reasons for not visiting, including the realities of distance and time involved. However, unconsciously, they may find it too painful to witness the decline of their parents. Or, unwittingly, they may be repaying parents for past unkindness or, more specifically, for lack of nurturing. It is only when we begin to understand what the past relationship has been, especially if the parent has been a difficult person to get along with, that we can free ourselves from blame. Then we can reduce our guilt feelings because we haven't done enough or because we resent that more is being asked of us.

"Conscience Doth Make Cowards of Us All"

When conscience accuses us unreasonably and makes us feel desirous of punishment for thoughts, fantasies, or actions, it also lowers our self-esteem. Feeling guilty is a feeling of blame. We blame ourselves when we experience a specific sense of personal failure, when we have disgraced our own view of what we think we ought to do or how we ought to behave. Then we are disappointed in ourselves.

101

MR. STACEY: "I really should know better. After all, I am a social worker. When my mother starts putting on her 'dependency act' and whines when I'm getting ready to leave after spending the weekend with her, I should just gently tell her, 'Mom, don't worry. I'll be back. I love you and everything will be okay because Aunt Margaret is here to take care of you.' But instead I get so wound up that I push her out of the way and insult her by calling her a baby. I guess that's the only way I can handle my guilt feelings.

"What do I feel guilty about? Probably because I'm not with her more often, and because I can't stand her needing me so much. When my father was alive, he took care of everything for her—she was treated like a princess. But, hell, my clients need me, too, and I need me. I'm afraid if I spread myself too thin I'll collapse."

When conscience is motivated and stimulated by our own internal standards of how we should behave, we feel guilty when we do not meet these standards. These internal standards are the goals we have for ourselves (our ego ideal) and the heights to which we aspire but may never reach. Mr. Stacey is a case in point.

Conscience may also be motivated by the fear of retaliation by an authority figure, usually a parent, sometimes God. The retaliation is for doing something wrong. Fear of losing our parents or fear of punishment also causes us to have guilty fear:

MS. ANN VETTER: "My father was in the hospital for almost four weeks with a kidney condition. While he was there he developed some bedsores, and one of them became infected. When it was time for him to be released, they were still treating the abscess on the bedsore. The dermatologist said that they never should have thought of releasing him so soon. But he'd been there so long!

"He was due to come home on Thursday, but his abscess was still draining. I had guilt feelings because—well, I wanted to go to a party on Saturday, but I knew I had to take Dad home. So I asked the doctor if he could keep him in the hospital until Sunday. And the doctor said they would release him on Monday, because the specialist had to be there and give instructions. But I had guilt feelings about keeping him in the hospital those extra days.

"Anyway, I did it, and I went to the party. Before I decided this, I told the doctor, 'Look, I have a party to go to.' He said, 'We'll keep him till Monday.' I said, 'Doctor, Monday is a holiday.' He said, 'All right, make it Tuesday morning.'

"The doctor seemed to think it was okay; he was a cooperative guy, that doctor. But, I also feel guilty because I went to the party and had a good time. I didn't even think of Dad until on the way home when I thought he would be angry with me if he knew where I had been."

Both these aspects of our conscience, guilt and guilty fear, contribute to our acts of kindness and caring toward others.

Guilt about Loss of Control

Family members often feel guilty when they become angry at the behavior of the person who is ill, even though they know the patient cannot control his behavior.

Ms. Jethro: "He keeps repeating over and over again: 'When do we eat, when do we eat, I'm hungry, when do we eat?' He'll say it a dozen or more times, after he just sat down and ate a sumptuous dinner that took me hours to prepare.

"I get so angry by the third time that I say something very mean and insulting to him, and sometimes I scream at the top of my lungs. Then I feel so guilty."

Feeling angry at such behavior is a normal response to frustration. The frustration is that the memory-impaired person does not respond to the preparations and feeding because he has no memory of the event. How insulting for the person not to remember you've spent hours shopping, cooking, preparing, and feeding him dinner. His question "When do we eat?" seems to wipe out the whole experience! When you react to

103

your frustrated feelings with anger, you're expressing a very human emotion. Still, we feel guilty about being so human:

Ms. Cohn: "The other night I lost my temper. I don't even remember what it was that upset me, but I scolded my poor Alfred. He has Alzheimer's disease, but he must have had a lucid moment when I was scolding him because he responded to my anger by saying, 'I don't think I belong here any more. I'm going to go away. I'm going to go out the door and go away and never come back.'

" 'Oh, Alfred, I didn't mean it. I'm so sorry.' I cried and then I kissed him. He forgot all about it, but I felt so guilty.

"After all, he's not capable of understanding, and it wasn't his fault anyway, but I was frustrated. I had to take it out on somebody and he was the only one there."

The fact that we want to provide care for our loved ones and we also care about them sometimes make us feel doubly resentful and upset at what they do. This may be because of our past relationship with them. The angry feelings may have nothing to do with the illness but may even go back five, ten, twenty years ago, or to when we were children and very competitive. We usually don't allow ourselves to feel those feelings because, if we did, we'd think, "My God, what kind of a monster am I that I should feel these feelings, when look at the terrible predicament my relative is in!"

Ms. Kincaid: "There are times when, try though I will to keep cool, I lose my composure and get terribly angry with my sister. I get so frustrated when she forgets what I told her just ten minutes ago. And while I'm screaming at her, it's a relief, but even so, I feel at the same time that I should shut up and stop screaming. . . . Because afterwards, I always have guilty feelings for having lost my temper.

"It's unfair of me to get angry at my sister. It's not her fault that she forgets. I ask myself, 'What if I were the one who had forgotten, would I want somebody to yell at me?' Of course not.

"But then I think maybe I'm angry at her for other things . . . things that happened when we were children. She always got everything first because she was older; I always had to wait and I hated it. But why should that matter now? That was so long ago."

Although feelings may get buried, they do not go away but stay suppressed until they find an avenue for expression through subtle humor, gentle teasing, or not so gentle but rather hostile attack. At times, our attacks may take place when the other person is at the lowest ebb in his life, or when some sickness or other debilitating event takes place, and then we can really let the other person have it. It's a form of "hitting below the belt." There may be some sadistic pleasure for Ms. Kincaid in seeing that once-powerful older sibling now helpless. Small wonder she feels guilty when she becomes aware of how she has misused her own power and, in essence, has taken advantage of her sister's weakened condition.

Most of the time, people like Ms. Kincaid have very little conscious awareness of what they are doing and do not seek to hurt their relative intentionally.

Guilt Shapes Generosity and Serves Society

Guilt is an emotion that shapes much of our goodness and generosity. Because guilt is such a discomforting emotion, it is much easier for us to feel anger than guilt. Therefore if something goes wrong, we tend to attribute that something to another person. We assign blame even when the other person was not at fault.

"If you hadn't upset me so with that awful remark about my sister, I wouldn't have burned your toast." We convert guilt into blame so quickly it's like handling a hot potato; we want to be rid of it in a big hurry. The wife who goes to the drugstore to pick up shaving cream for her husband, then loses her purse on the way home, blames him: "You and your stupid shaving cream!"

If a spouse or a parent delays calling for help for much longer than is wise, or if the caregiver fails to recognize the need for that help before it is asked for, whom shall we blame? In the case of the spouse or parent, we tend to blame the victim for refusing medical care (or perhaps for dangerous driving, smoking, or drinking). In the case of the caregiver, we blame ourselves. There is a feeling in both of these situations that a catastrophe need never have occurred; we become angry at the victim and at ourselves.

Guilt helps us to serve society, on whose members we are dependent for our survival. No human being can live without the nurturance of other human beings. More nurturing in the form of loving and caring enhances our own sense of humanity. When we are given less nurturing, our sense of humanity is diminished. Thus guilt fuses the individual to the group. Similarly, guilt and its companion emotions—pity, shame, caring, loving compassion, and empathy—bind us to those upon whom we depend for our survival and those who depend upon us in order to survive, including the victims of Alzheimer's disease or other chronic illnesses.

If we detect so much as a small impulse of hatred toward a loved one, we usually are very concerned about it and feel guilty. These are such painful feelings that we try very hard to disguise or refrain from feeling them. However, the feelings become a source of discomfort when, even in disguise, they interfere with relationships between people. The distress we experience when we feel unappreciated (even by a stranger) tends to come from unconscious feelings of unworthiness of the regard of others. A cold reception from someone may confirm our own suspicions of our unworthiness. Dissatisfaction with our appearance, our work, or any of our abilities leads us to feel inferior. Feelings of this kind are connected with unconscious feelings of guilt. People who need constant praise and approval have a need for continual evidence that they are worthy of being loved and that they are lovable. The underlying fear is that they are incapable of truly loving others. More particularly, if they are unable to master their feelings of aggression toward a loved one, they dread being a source of danger to that person. When the feelings run deep and are repressed for a long time, the caregiver may become verbally or physically abusive to the victim, as in the case of Michaela Cardena:

"I am very, very frightened about my behavior. My grandmother has become worse and my tolerance has become minimal.

"My grandmother is constantly talking. The more anxious she becomes, the more she babbles. I'm ashamed to describe what happened today when she began jabbering. I asked her to please be quiet, but she just kept it up. I guess she doesn't understand what 'Please be quiet' means anymore. Then I begged her: '*Please* don't talk!' Then I shouted: 'PLEASE—BE QUIET!' I told her in Spanish to keep quiet, or, literally, 'Shut up.' When I heard my own words, I knew I was being ugly. This is the woman who raised me when my own mother died. She is somebody I love, she's been like a mother to me. But when she wouldn't stop babbling, I just took my hand and clasped it over her mouth—'PLEASE stop it!' I yelled, and I was almost hysterical. I hate myself for it, and I feel so guilty.

"It's ugly, and I know I'm being abusive. When I covered her mouth like that, she lost her balance and fell, and she hit her head on the wall. Suddenly I saw blood on the floor. I tried to tell myself, 'Stay calm—it's nothing. She's fine, she's fine, stay calm.' I picked her up, quietly, and I put her on the toilet seat. There was blood running out of her nose. The sight of the blood sobered me immediately. That really made me feel sick. 'What a stinking person you are! You're really ugly, Michaela!' I told myself.

"I got an ice pack and put it on her nose, and tried to put some cotton in it, and she FOUGHT! She kept pulling my hands away all the time I was trying to put the cotton in. As soon as I had it in, she pulled it out.

"Then I got angry at her again. 'I'm trying to help you. I'm your granddaughter, I'm trying to help you!' And she kept screaming and carrying on, and I'm sure that the neighbors, by now, think that the grandchild is killing her grandmother, or at the very least is abusing her physically.

"Finally I calmed her. Then I became very loving, and I said, 'I'm sorry—you're nice. You're a nice lady, you're a nice lady.' (Of course, I'll probably lash out at her again, another time.) She got very docile, and we were genuinely affectionate with each other. I really felt awful about this display of anger. I have terrible anger. I have such rage that I'm terrified of it. I felt so guilty about her bloody nose, I wasn't going to go to my support group meeting. But then I realized how much I need to tell people how I really feel, so I went."

Balanced by your concern and caring for the patient, frustration, anger, and guilt are merely part of a total emotional relationship. Try to remember how many nurturing and selfless efforts you have made on behalf of the patient; perhaps then you won't be so devastated by any angry or hostile feelings. Then you won't feel so guilty. Remorse and guilt are exaggerated when other family members and friends respond to the chronically ill, memory-impaired patient by ostracizing him. Are they afraid the illness is contagious? No, memory impairment is usually not contagious, but some family members may fear becoming like the forgetful person. Others may be uncertain as to how to respond to the patient. "What should I say when Aunt Sally asks who I am? I'm afraid I'll giggle. I always giggle when I'm nervous." This was a comment by a fifteen-year-old niece exposed to her aunt during an infrequent visit to the nursing home.

As invitations, visits, and phone calls inevitably decrease when there is a chronically ill patient, the family caregiver may feel blamed and punished by other family members or friends.

Conscious Guilt about Practical Considerations

NANCY CROSSMAN: "Lisa and I first met when we taught in a small prep school in Illinois. The first year we shared a house for economy's sake, but during that year we discovered a love as true and as beautiful as any married couple ever felt. We decided to live together permanently; that was over forty years ago. We shared our money in a joint account and built a summer house together.

"Since Lisa become ill, twelve years ago, I've taken care of her. I feed her and dress her and pay all her bills.

"I have finally taken all the money from our joint account and opened one small savings account in her own name because she gave me power of attorney years ago. I don't know if it's right. Legally, I don't have responsibility for her because I'm not a blood relative. There is almost no law which relates to a common-law homosexual marriage. I know I'm the one who is caring for her, and yet I still feel guilty about what might look to others like I was taking her money. No matter what I do I feel guilty.

"When I talk about this problem to friends, even though they agree with what I'm doing, I find myself describing my actions in ways that will make me look praiseworthy and honorable. I want them to continue to think well of me.

"We made wills leaving everything to each other, but I feel guilty. If she dies, I guess her body will be 'mine,' too, and I would like to give her brain to science for autopsy. It will help us all learn more about Lisa's disease. But she was always a religious person, and I'm not sure whether she would approve of that action.

"I haven't talked to a lawyer, either about that or about my legal responsibilities in terms of our money, because I feel that by talking to a lawyer, I'm taking the first step down the road to getting rid of her, and that makes me feel guilty, too."

Ms. Crossman expresses the feelings of many friends and relatives who must get power of attorney in order to administer the business affairs of their spouse, parent, or other person with whom they are living.

There is a sense of guilt even about practical matters, such as making sure the impaired person's finances are made available for his continued care.

Guilt about finances may have its roots in a couple's earliest relationship with respect to money. In many traditional households where the husband is the major breadwinner and the wife is a homemaker, it is customary that he makes major financial decisions; in more democratic households, joint tenancy in stocks and bonds and joint savings and checking accounts are the custom. Where the husband's role is more autocratic, some wives are fearful of their husband's ire if he should find out that she now controls the purse strings.

A case in point is the Maleskis. Gena and Max are from the "old school." She rules the roost, and he rules the outside world and their finances. When Max started to become ill, Gena joined a support group. She complained to the group that the bank would frequently call to say that Max had forgotten to sign or endorse his checks. Gradually, his numbers became unclear, then his handwriting become illegible, and finally his signature became hardly recognizable. At this point Gena, at the urging of other group members who had already had this experience with their own relatives, went to the branch bank manager and told him that her husband was ill and losing his memory.

She had previously gotten Max to sign over a power of attorney by telling him to practice his signature on the piece of paper she placed in front of him. Gena was now able to sign checks for the rent, telephone, and all their expenses. It wasn't easy for her to take over this job because it was unfamiliar to her, but at the prompting of her accountant and her son she managed to do it.

But when one day, unbeknownst to Gena, Max went to the bank and had his check refused, Gena panicked. All of the guilt she had not been expressing surfaced. Max accused her of taking his money; Gena felt criminal and, indeed, behaved as if she were a thief. "It's his money," she cried, "he worked hard for it; now he can't even write a check for $10.00. I did the wrong thing."

Until Gena realized that Max didn't really know what he was saying, and that he accused her unjustly, she felt enormously guilty. She failed to remember that she told Max she would pay all the bills from now on to make it easier for him, and that he had smiled and said nothing, almost silently agreeing that it was best for everybody.

Perhaps she was feeling guilty because of how she had gained the power of attorney. Duping Max into signing the power of attorney agreement was what troubled her the most. She hated to do it that way, but she felt there was no alternative. Somebody had to look out for them, so it had to be Gena.

Helping Gena to realize all of this took time and effort, but with the support from others who had gone through similar or worse experiences, Gena was able to feel better about what she had done. Talking about her fears and guilty feelings with the group psychotherapist enabled Gena to diminish them; after a while she was no longer troubled by guilt over her behavior.

Guilt over Institutionalization

MRS. SWOBODA: "I've been married for forty-five years. You can't ignore that; you can't cut it out. That's what's holding me back from finding a nursing home. Even if my husband were in a home, I wouldn't be at peace. My mind would be there with him, anyway, and I'd go to see him every day.

"There's that gnawing guilt feeling. Put it any way you want, there's that guilt. You see, I get so angry with him I could almost kill him, and then I catch myself and I say, 'What the hell am I thinking? He's my dear husband. The marriage vows said, 'For better or for worse, in sickness and in health.'

"But his sickness is killing me. I can't lift him anymore to put him on the toilet. I'm worn out. When I think about putting him away I feel so guilty. Would he do that if I was the one who got sick? I feel so criminal for even thinking about a nursing home. But, he's getting worse . . . "

MR. NICKERSON: "I'm so guilty, guilty, guilty. Even though I took care of her for six years—washed her, bathed her, took her to the toilet, cared for her, and was loving and tender to her until she got so unmanageable that I had to put her in the hospital. She had such outbursts that she fell on the floor and I thought she was foaming at the mouth. I had to get a neighbor in to help me pick her up. So we took her to the hospital and she's been there two weeks.

"I can't look her in the eye. When I go to visit her, sometimes she doesn't even know who I am. But I feel guilty because now I have to put her away in a nursing home. She was always a good woman, a kind woman, gentle, loving, caring. We had our fights, but we always made up. Our son died twelve years ago; a few years later I got very sick with colitis, and she took care of me as if I were her little boy. Nothing was

111

too good for me. She catered to me and helped me to get well. Yes, I took care of her, too, but now. . . .

"I feel so guilty. I'm afraid she's thinking that I'm deserting her. . . . I wonder if she can still think?"

Some of Mr. Nickerson's guilt is provoked by his yearning for freedom from the endless pressure of providing continual care for his wife. For the past two weeks he's had more freedom than in the six years of his wife's illness. Even though he misses his wife, he's enjoying not having to put diapers on her or having to pick up after her. But he feels that he has abandoned her when she needs him so much.

Mr. Nickerson's concern is that he is behaving badly by deserting his wife. He is being self-critical. The guilt he is experiencing is that of separation.

As we grow up, we develop a unique personality by identifying with and imitating the most important people in our lives (mother and father). Unconsciously we internalize aspects of our mother's and father's personality into our own. Gradually we become our own independent and unique personality.

Mr. Nickerson explained that he had never really separated from his mother. He was her only son and youngest child and lived at home throughout his school years, acting as her "man of the house" until the day he was married. Then he became "the man of the house" to his wife. Mr. Nickerson, who had often been sickly as a child, had been very emotionally dependent on his mother. Later he transferred that dependency to his wife. They did everything together. He had been trained as a lawyer, and for most of their married life he used the extra bedroom in the house for his office, so he was even at home during the day. They were able, far more than most families, to share equally in the day-to-day aspects of raising their children.

When their son died, Mr. Nickerson experienced feelings of isolation from his wife for the first time since their marriage. Neither husband nor wife could comfort the other; neither parent mourned openly. Instead, Mr. Nickerson became ill, ironically, with the same disease that had killed his son. But he was lucky—doctors were able to operate before peritonitis developed. His wife nursed him back to health. A few years later Mrs. Nickerson developed Alzheimer's disease. Mr. Nickerson has not developed sufficient ego strength to face the rest of his life alone. He suffers from separation anxiety, which gives rise to feelings of guilt at the thought of being a mature and independent person.

What can he do about it? First of all, he must recognize that he feels guilty. After he has taken that first step, talking about his feelings with an empathic psychotherapist or counselor will help him to understand where his feelings of guilt come from. As he begins the therapeutic process, he will be able to understand the past and then recognize that, while he cannot change the past, he can have control over his future. As he comes to understand and feel less guilty, some of his embarrassment about his wife's "odd" behavior will dissipate. Guilt over not always treating his wife kindly and courteously, and for getting angry at her while she is helpless and ill, minor guilt over yelling at her, major guilt for putting her in the nursing home and now not wanting her to return home—all will be admitted, understood, and worked through emotionally. "She made me feel guilty," he cried. "She said if I loved her I would be more compassionate when she couldn't find the word she wanted (she had always been a good reader and a lively and colorful conversationalist with a precise use of language). Her condition is getting worse and worse. Should I have done more for her, talked to her more, given her more love and affection? Sometimes I just don't want the responsibility for her any more, and then do I feel guilty!"

Mr. Nickerson has many guilty feelings with which he needs to come to terms. Some of these are over small matters like forgetting to do something for his wife that she liked—a "sin of omission"; others are for equally small or serious acts that are "sins of commission" (actually doing something when the consequences lead to injuring or hurting the feelings of another person). Still more deep-seated is the separation anxiety that Mr. Nickerson feels. It may imply to him that he is rejecting his wife, abandoning her so that he can get on with his life and the many options he feels are now open to him. But unless he works through these more substantial reasons for feeling guilty, he will not be able to use any of these options. He will feel too guilty to enjoy himself and may even feel that he needs to be punished for wanting to give up his responsibility and have something gratifying and uniquely his, for himself alone.

How many times, in their younger and healthier years, have husbands, wives, children, and friends vowed never to institutionalize one another? At the time the promise was made, it was meant to be kept. However, circumstances change, and we may be forced to alter our plans to celebrate our golden years together, even to the point of having to break a sacred promise never to institutionalize a loved one.

Mrs. Rowenbach sat tearfully in a group therapy session clutching her handkerchief. For five months she had been wrestling with her ambivalent feelings about putting her husband in a nursing home.

In his lucid moments, Mr. Rowenbach reminded his wife of her promise never to put him in a home. Only 62 and still handsome, although he walks with a stooped gait and shuffling feet, he's become incontinent both from the bladder and the anus. Mrs. Rowenbach can't tolerate it, even though she has paid to keep nurses' aides around the clock. "Sometimes he's very abusive to me," she says, "and even though I know he doesn't mean it, I cringe. The tranquilizers make him like a zombie. It's like living with a ghost. He frightens me."

Because Mrs. Rowenbach was wearing herself out physically and emotionally, the group therapist had been trying to help her make the decision to put her husband in a nursing home. Mrs. Rowenbach remained uncertain. While, on the one hand, she felt very guilty about breaking her word, on the other hand, she wanted to do what was best both for her husband and for herself.

The psychotherapist offered to make the decision for her, if that would help. But the therapist emphasized, at the same time, that to accept the decision-making of others was to avoid both her own responsibility and coping with her guilt.

After several more sessions, Mrs. Rowenbach realized that *she* would have to make the decision, not her therapist, or her children, or her wish to be guided by the past. In the present, she bore the pain of the guilt, made the decision, and carried it out effectively.

Some months later she told the therapist that what was instrumental in helping her make her own decision was the recognition that, indeed, she would have liked someone else to take that responsibility away from her; it would exonerate her from the pain of her guilt feelings. She is working these through now and is able to see that she made the correct choice. There are no regrets. It is painful, but she is surviving well and feels more comfortable with herself now. By remaining actively involved in her husband's care in the nursing home, Mrs. Rowenbach is able to reduce her sense of guilt. She is also recognizing that she needs a certain amount of freedom for herself, and although this knowledge is guilt-provoking, the therapist and the group are providing support for the expression and fulfillment of her needs. The support is essential to helping her reduce her anxiety and depression.

Even as caregivers try to avoid it, for some people institutionalization is inevitable as the progressive deterioration of Alzheimer's disease runs its course and takes it toll, both on the victim and the caregiver.

Caregivers like Mrs. Rowenbach are hard put to break their solemn pledges; they suffer great guilt and remorse when this is necessary. Feeling helpless, vanquished, and without hope, few caregivers recognize that institutionalization may be the ultimate act of love toward the patient. When the caregiver has reached the limits of his emotional and financial resources, unburdening himself of the loved one is an act of kindness to oneself and the patient. It is an act of love that can free the caregiver to provide more sustenance for himself and thereby, albeit indirectly, for the person who is ill. If we cannot love ourselves and be compassionate to our own needs, how can we possibly nourish or be of comfort to another?

Guilt is difficult to dissipate. Like a nagging pain, it can become a constant companion that plagues family members and causes them to be especially hard on themselves. Recognizing that you've done the best you can with the intellectual knowledge you possess and your own emotional resources is one way to keep from blaming yourself. The patient's illness and his failure to respond more hopefully to your loving care and thoughtful concern is not your fault.

Guilty because you are insecure, because parents, spouse, boss, or friends fail to appreciate your qualities, loved ones put you down, and you feel depleted in your self-esteem? A good antidote to feeling guilty is to repeat several times: "I'm a decent person," "I'm doing the best I can," "I'm not guilty." Stick to this belief, and don't let anyone manipulate or intimidate you into feeling guilty. Remember, also, that most people feel guilty at times for things where guilt is unjustified.

Talking about your guilt feelings with a good friend or an empathic psychotherapist is extremely helpful and will relieve you of the burden of that uncomfortable emotion.

CHAPTER 9

Fears: Present and Future

Ms. Anna Jean tearfully entered the therapy room after a one-week hiatus. She had gone to visit her mother in Missouri. Mother had been diagnosed as having Alzheimer's disease nine months previously. It had been a shock to the entire family.

"But she's so young," cried Ms. Jean, as she grabbed tissues from the holder and blew her nose. Her mother was only 51 years old. Ms. Jean, a young, vibrant 22-year-old, had gone to New York two years before to pursue a dancing career. Beautiful and talented, she was having some emotional difficulties adjusting to the demands of her career, and there were problems with her boyfriend, whom she knew from college. He was also in the arts, a talented musician trying to get a recording contract for his rock band.

It was evident that in this last visit home, Ms. Jean was shaken by her mother's somewhat strange and erratic behavior. Mother had always been flamboyant and outgoing. While she recognized her daughter, smiling and welcoming her home, at times she became frozen in her expressions, didn't remember her daughter's name, and ordered the nursing aide out of the home. Ms. Jean's father had lost weight and was undone by his wife's diagnosis. He had leaned heavily on her all of his life, but now the roles were reversed; he was the major caregiver.

"I'm so afraid," Ms. Jean cried. "My mother is not herself and never will be again. In the past five months since I saw her, she's gotten much worse. I can't bear to look at her. Everytime I see her, I remember how beautiful she was; her clothes were always immaculate, and she never had a hair out of place." Ms. Jean's mother had been a dynamic woman who helped her daughter cultivate an interest in dance; since her childhood her mother had taken Ms. Jean for dancing lessons and to dance recitals.

Ms. Jean was not just sad because of her mother's illness and her feelings of helplessness; she had discussed these feelings in previous sessions. Now there was fear on the face of this young woman. She spoke about the fear of the possibility of it happening to her—fear of becoming a victim of Alzheimer's disease.

Ms. Jean discussed her anxiety with her sister Tina, who lived near their mother, but found no comfort. For Tina, seeing the daily deterioration of her mother brought on other fears: that her mother would hurt herself, that her care would be inadequate, and that she faced many years in a condition she hated.

Anna and Tina Jean are not alone; everyone close to victims of Alzheimer's disease must wrestle with fears. Often these anxieties remain unspoken; sometimes people don't even recognize them in their minds. This is especially true of the fear that one might develop Alzheimer's disease oneself, a fear that doesn't usually surface until the patient is in the late stages of the illness. For Ms. Anna Jean, her identification with her mother's plight came early because of their closeness and because she still felt a need for mothering.

It is very important to recognize the anxieties brought on by Alzheimer's disease. Otherwise, your mind can unconsciously protect itself by shielding you from the trigger for those anxieties, the patient. Fears can first become manifest when friends and relatives neglect to visit the patient. People may find "good reasons" to stay away: their own families, work, the long trip, and so on. Caregivers may choose not to take certain steps, like talking to nursing homes, because such actions would acknowledge the severity of the patient's illness. It is important to deal with your fears, to do as much as you reasonably can to alleviate them, and to move on—both for the patient and for yourself.

In the rest of this chapter we discuss fears that caregivers commonly express and how you can overcome them.

Fear of Letting a Patient Hurt Himself

Caregivers are often unaware of the necessity for increasing attentiveness to keep an Alzheimer's victim from harm until an accident occurs. The patient may hurt himself by mistaking an artificial fruit or an artificial flower for edible food. He may open the door to the basement, forget to look, and fall down the basement stairs. One patient walked through an open gate and landed in the swimming pool. Others have stepped out into the road in the midst of traffic. There have been reports of patients cutting themselves with knives and scalding themselves with boiling water they couldn't feel (sensations of hot and cold are often lost). Others have eaten poisonous things in the fields behind their houses. The list of possible dangers to Alzheimer's victims is long and unfortunately too real.

How the caregiver can deal with the real dangers of ordinary household living is covered in Chapter 12. Here we address the fear of caregivers that these things *can* happen. Obviously, the best solution is to take preventive steps and "adult-proof" the house to keep the person from harm. Prepare for the worst *before* the patient reaches that stage.

Make the house as safe as possible, but don't sit and worry about accidents; they can and do happen. If an accident occurs, don't be alarmed. Try to remain cool and give your patient as much tenderness and kindness as you can muster at the moment. Afterwards, don't blame yourself; focus on keeping that danger from reappearing, and be proud that you have taken a positive action.

Fear of Hurting a Patient Emotionally

"We always hurt the one we love," is an old refrain. Caregivers often fear they will hurt their patients by being too strict or emotional with them. Showing annoyance, frustration, or anger will probably upset the

119

patient, but he will soon forget the hurt. It's best that you forget the incident, too. In trying circumstances even the best of us can hurt the ones we love.

Don't try to hold in your anger because it will come out in other ways. Remember the words of the poet William Blake:

> *I was angry at my friend.*
> *I told my wrath, and it did end.*
> *I was angry with my foe.*
> *I told it not, my wrath did grow.*

Tell the patient if you are angry with him, or with the disease. He may be able to sense your emotion only from the tone of your voice and probably will not remember why you are upset. But tell him anyway to relieve your own tension.

If you find yourself repeatedly hurting a patient by handling him too roughly, seek counseling immediately. You are probably trying to unconsciously work out some of your negative feelings. Both you and the patient deserve help with this issue.

Ms. Jarrett, a 48-year-old caregiver who herself was a psychotherapist, sought counseling to help her to deal with her fears of hurting her 74-year-old mother, who was a victim of Alzheimer's disease.

"She's always been such a good mother to me, a kind and caring, sensitive lady with a good sense of humor," explained Ms. Jarrett. "When I comb her hair, I think of how I felt as a child when she combed my hair. She would praise me and say I was pretty and would have good fortune in my life. Humph!—some good fortune. Look at me now, taking care of my own mother who is now like a child."

The resentment in her tone was loud and clear to me, although until it was gently pointed out, Ms. Jarrett was not aware of it. She still wanted to be the child of her loving mother, so once in a while she "unconsciously" gave a tug at the old woman's hair. It was not malicious, just a way of expressing how unlucky she felt. After all, Ms. Jarrett was taking care of her own patients and was in a sense a mother to them. Now the roles were reversed with her own mother, whom she had to mother.

Some people welcome the prospect of nurturing elders as a continuation of the life cycle. For others who still feel the need for nurturing themselves, it is an unwanted task.

After several sessions, Ms. Jarrett began to realize that she so enjoyed the warmth and closeness she had always had with her mother that it was very painful to give up being "fed" by her and learning to take responsibility for herself.

When motives for caregiving are honest, we can forgive ourselves the imperfect attunement we may at times display to others. All we can hope for is to be "good enough" caregivers. After all, no one is perfect. We do err, make mistakes, have moments of doubt, get upset, and remain vulnerable to the emotional vicissitudes that caring for such a patient can induce.

Fear of Being Hurt

Caregivers who have experienced catastrophic reactions with their Alzheimer's patients often fear for their own safety. Sometimes a patient can become enraged seemingly without provocation. He may berate the caregiver or accuse him of doing away with his spouse or stealing his money. The patient may ask for his mother or a long departed relative and then become very agitated. Some patients have threatened caregivers or abused them verbally. Others have pushed and shoved them violently or threatened them with a weapon! It is important for caregivers to note that getting out of the line of fire is the most important step in taking charge of the situation. Don't try to physically restrain the patient unless you are a judo or karate expert and can handle the enormous physical strength that can be evidenced by the patient. You may have to enlist the aid of a trained police expert to help you.

Eventually the patient will calm down. Later he will become docile, almost angelic, and will not be aware of any of the damage he's done. He can't apologize or soothe your feelings or even notice that you have feelings about anything. For the Alzheimer's patient, the incident is over. Was it provoked by something real that you said or did, or did it

121

come from the unconscious? The patient cannot tell you. But if it's over, let it be over!

Try to deal with your own feelings by doing a relaxation exercise, performing mental visualization, meditating, or getting out and doing something physical to relieve your tension. You might also try to "breathe your stress away." Take deep breaths for five seconds from the diaphragm, and then let your breath out slowly, making a slight hissing sound. Then add a sigh, yawn, grunt, groan, or moan, using all the techniques of breathing. You'll be able to breathe through your fears, anxieties, and frustrations. Breathing raises the endorphin levels in your brain. These endorphins are natural painkiller substances (like morphine) that can lower your blood pressure and heart rate and calm you down when you are under any stress. We all have to learn how to handle our own anger. Otherwise, it eats us up alive, interferes with our loving feelings, and creates havoc in our relationships. Reread Chapter 6 to help you with this difficult emotion.

Shame Is a Special Fear

Shame is anger about what should not be. In a child, shame threatens his survival; in an adult with Alzheimer's disease, shaming the victim for behavior out of his control leads to his fear of abandonment by the caregiver on whom he is dependent.

Everyone at different moments in life experiences shame about some aspect of themselves. The everyday consequences of shame can be a major source of human misery and suffering.

Shame and embarrassment have much in common. They are often felt simultaneously. Shame is a painful experience in which the sense of the self is diminished. Embarrassment can be equally painful, but it also can be an emotionally trivial experience or even a partially pleasant experience. When we are embarrassed, we're thrown off kilter, an uncomfortable state to be in. We feel rattled and off-balance, and our composure is disrupted. Embarrassment can become shame when it is clearly linked to a negative idea about the self or to a negative self-perception.

The loss of control over mental functions and emotions may elicit shame in the Alzheimer's patient. He may be ashamed of his loss of memory because he feels diminished. After all, memory is what keeps us connected to our feelings about people and events. When we cannot confidently interact with people, remembering the joys we've shared or the environment we live in, we become disappointed. We've failed ourselves in terms of our self-image or ego ideal. The Alzheimer's patient feels inferior and defective. An intense sense of displeasure overtakes him and he wishes to be restored—to be more intact, to feel whole, not to be confused, to have his memory back. He does not feel worthwhile or good enough. It is a conviction of being flawed and incompetent even though the incompetence is the result of illness. The patient feels humiliated because he's been put into a lowered or degraded position. He may blame himself for this humiliated status. Ultimately self-blame and self-loathing foster low self-esteem and create depression. Shame may play a larger role in depression than does guilt.

For the caregiver, however, the shame that comes from embarrassment over the Alzheimer's patient's plight in life, as well as over his peculiar habits and behavior, can become a chronic feeling that sours everyday life and its activities. The caregiver may direct his bitterness and animosity toward himself as he realizes the futility of his efforts to restore the patient to a former state of mental functioning and emotional well-being.

It is only through genuine understanding and friendship that these kinds of shameful feelings can be healed. Indeed, in small doses, shame can lead to self-improvement, self-discovery, and a healthy willingness to examine those things about ourselves that make us feel bad. Perhaps then we can constructively and reasonably change them.

When the Patient Needs More Help

Many caregivers are able to cope emotionally, physically, and financially with an Alzheimer's victim who is manageable at home. But there is always the lurking fear about what happens when it gets worse. Then the family has to employ outside help, such as home health aides. The possibility of not being able to care for the patient at home arises. The expense of such care is a related source of fear and anxiety. These are all real fears that must be explored and are best dealt with in counseling, either individually or in a professionally run support group. Subsequent chapters will address some of these questions more fully.

Caregivers may also fear what will happen to the patient if they suffer an illness or accident. Contingency plans are always very important to consider and are discussed in Chapter 14.

The Silent Question

Will I get it? That is the unspoken question on the lips of the children of Alzheimer's patients. How can one assure them that they won't become victims of this terrible scourge? Alzheimer's disease is not contagious, but there is a genetic factor. We look to statistics for some measure of comfort. Our current knowledge tells us that not all forms of Alzheimer's disease are inherited. Children of Alzheimer's patients have only a 10 to 20 percent greater chance than the general population of developing the illness. However, we also know that Alzheimer's disease does run in some families.

The risk of developing Alzheimer's disease is less than 1 percent before the age of 50 but increases rapidly in each successive decade of life. It reaches 30 percent by age 90. Where there is familial Alzheimer's disease, immediate family relatives have a 50 percent chance of developing Alzheimer's disease sometime during their lives because the tendency is transmitted as a dominant trait.

SHOULD PEOPLE LIVE IN FEAR OF GETTING ALZHEIMER'S DISEASE?

Living with the fear of getting Alzheimer's disease—or any other illness, for that matter—can curtail the freedom and spontaneity of life that helps people to put their creative energies into living. Becoming a dancer or a painter, a businessperson or a lawyer, a nurse or a teacher, a clerical worker or a mother, requires faith in one's ability to perform the physical and mental labors that constitute our basic "job descriptions."

Fear is a stressor, a killer that not only inhibits life but detracts from one's ability to live. In and of itself, fear can debilitate the human psyche and produce physical, mental, and emotional symptomatology that can lead to physical and emotional illness. The fears of parents are visited upon their children, preventing them from growing up to be strong and independent.

A fearful child often becomes an anxiety-ridden, neurotic adult incapable of caring for himself in the best possible way. Without the help of a competent psychotherapist, these adults may perpetuate a lifetime of unnecessary strife and grief.

Fear of "Living Death"

We have not discussed patients' fears because victims of advanced Alzheimer's disease are not able to express them verbally. In the early stage of the illness, some people can talk about their fears of further deterioration and concerns for their own safety. Others mention their fear of being unable to continue providing for dependent relatives.

The caregiver can discuss such anxieties with the patient early in the illness. As difficult as that conversation may be, you can reassure the patient that he and his loved ones will be cared for. Discuss plans for the future, such as how the patient wants his estate handled and whether he wishes to be kept alive by extraordinary medical means. The patient may not be able to have this discussion; offer him options to which he can say "yes" or "no."

SUICIDE AND EUTHANASIA

Is suicide always an act of temporary insanity? Or can it be the act of a rational person aware of what looms in front of him: physical decline, mental deterioration, loss of friendships, isolation, and ultimately, loss

125

of self? There are few statistics about suicide among people with Alzheimer's disease. It is my belief, somewhat controversial still, that suicide can be a rational act by someone considering the quality of his life and what makes life meaningful.

For an Alzheimer's patient, suicide can only be considered rational if it is done at the onset of the illness, when the patient still has the mental ability to make such a decision. The Alzheimer's victim is at some level *always* aware of his loss of memory and loss of function and is concerned for his safety, even though he cannot verbalize such feelings. As the disease progresses, he might ask for assistance to die, from either a loved one or a physician, or even a nurse or aide. Providing such assistance constitutes euthanasia, or "mercy killing," in its more popular terminology. The purpose of euthanasia is to end the endless suffering of the victim by either helping him to commit suicide or ending his life for him. Euthanasia is a highly charged subject, since it involves moral and religious principles as well as legal issues. However, the newspapers are filled with more and more accounts: a physician in Michigan who helped his patient to die via a "death machine," a husband in Florida who could no longer bear the suffering of his wife and killed her with a shotgun.

These are the more sensational accounts that we read about in the newspapers or hear about on television. What we don't hear about are the "little murders" that are probably more routine: when caregivers neglect or forget to give medications, when family members neglect to call or visit, when formerly loving friends turn away. Society turns its back on Alzheimer's victims and their families by participating in their financial ruin through the improper demand that families impoverish themselves before the state or federal government will take over the financial burden of caring for the patients. These actions produce much anguish, frustration, and bitterness that might be alleviated by a change in society's attitudes toward chronic illness and Alzheimer's disease.

Whose life is it anyway: God's, the family's, society's, or the patient's? What if the patient is mentally incompetent? Why can't we help patients to die with dignity? Should the physician withhold treatment that seems to prolong the dying process when the patient will never regain the ability to make decisions and express his wishes? If the patient is conscious, does he have the right to tell his physician that he does not want cardiac resuscitation, tube feeding, or mechanical respiration, or antibiotics? These questions become dilemmas in the face of society's moral and ethical repulsion toward suicide. The traditional tenet is that all human life is equally valuable. We must focus, however, on the *quality* of human life rather than the sanctity of human life. Is it humane or rational to preserve life when circumstances such as age or pain or terminal illness suggest the burdens of life outweigh the benefits?

Your life is your own. It belongs to no one else, and you make of your life what you can, given the circumstances of your birth and environmental advantages. If you have come to terms rationally, before any disease process occurs, with the meaning of life and how you want to live it, taking your life through suicide is your sole responsibility. The sharing of that act via euthanasia by significant people in your life, who know and share your views, ideas, and feelings, is a true act of devotion!

Preparing a Living Will

To consider the patient's wishes, we must first be aware of them. He must make his wishes known. Appendix C is an example of a living will. This document is a voluntary declaration by the patient of his request that medical personnel refrain from life-sustaining procedures that artificially prolong the dying process. This declaration, along with a durable power of attorney for health care, should be signed by the patient at the outset of his illness so that there is no misunderstanding about how he wants to complete his life.

The question arises as to when it is rational for a person to commit suicide. At the outset of Alzheimer's disease, a person can still enjoy certain aspects of life. No one can make the decision as to when life becomes unbearable but the Alzheimer's victim himself. Perhaps when he feels he is too personally burdened by his illness he will not be able to make the decision. Probably then the decision has to be made right away, with specific directions being given to loved ones if he is enlisting their aid. A group known as Choice In Dying can be very helpful to

127

Alzheimer's victims and also to the families of patients who have not expressed a wish. Through their literature and through counseling, they can help people with their decision-making process. Other helpful organizations are listed in Appendix A.

What profits us to continue a life in a vegetative state that can know no sound of music, no feel of wind, no smell of a rose, no memory of past loves, no feeling of present joy, but only pain, anguish, suffering, and fear, with only more of the same to look forward to each day? That is a living death, not life. Releasing the spirit of the Alzheimer's victim from the diseased brain is an act of human kindness. I believe that God will forgive this act and the soul will not suffer because of it.

Brief Guidelines to Recognizing and Identifying Your Feelings

You are feeling:	When you say:
Ambivalent	"I can't stand taking care of her anymore. It's unbearable. Maybe I'll walk out on her . . . but I can't—she was such a loving wife to me until she got sick."
Anxious	"I always come about an hour early when we have an appointment. I don't like to be late."
Ashamed	"Everytime I lose my temper at my father because he forgets, I hate myself."
Confused	"I'd like to get a job, but I really don't know what to do."
Depressed (moderately)	"I can't concentrate on the newspaper or television." Or, "I wish I were away from it all."
Depressed (severely)	"I can't sleep, I have no appetite, and I've lost weight. I'm so tired, and I constantly have constipation (or diarrhea)."
Deserted	"I am lost. My sister is dead; I have no close friends."
Despairing	"I have no one who cares about me; life is not worth living."
Disappointed	"I was so proud of my granddaughter until this happened. I can't believe she did a thing like that."
Distrustful	"The doctors don't tell me everything, I know. They tell my children what's wrong with me."
Embarrassed	"I'd like to talk about the problem, but I was raised to keep such things private."
Empathic	"I understand the way you feel."

129

Fearful	"My memory is not as good as it used to be. Maybe I'll take the wrong bus."
Frustrated	"I've told you ten times already, it's summer and you don't need to wear a coat."
Guilty (for real acts)	"I am guilty because I yelled at my father when he was ill."
Guilty (for imagined acts)	"I should have helped my children more."
Guilt (for past failures)	
—over errors	"I made a mistake when I quit that job."
—over indiscretions	"It was unwise to tell Maggie about Jim's affair."
Helpless	"There is nothing I can do about my situation. Things will never change."
Hopeless	"Now that the kids don't need me, my life has no meaning anymore."
Hurt	"My son wants to spend the Easter holidays with his in-laws; he always spent them with me."
Inadequate	"I don't know how to have fun anymore."
Insulted	"Why did you take away the keys to my car?"
Intimate	"We can tell each other how we feel when we're well and when we're sick. It's been that way for a long time."
Jealous	"She always gets visitors on Mother's Day, Christmas, Easter, and every Sunday. I don't."
Joyful	"It's been so long since my son has visited me. I'm looking forward to it."
Lonely	"I don't talk to a human being all day. I leave the television blaring just so I can hear human voices." "I don't believe in God."
Mature love	"We don't have to be glued together to love each other."
Misunderstood	"My daughter doesn't approve of the new man in my life."

Peaceful	"There is only one life here on earth, and I'm content with how I've lived my life."
Regretful	"My mother is dying, and I haven't gone to see her. We haven't really had anything to say to each other for years. Now that she's dying, I feel awful. I don't want her to die with things the way they are between us now."
Relieved	"We talked about those old misunderstandings and settled them. It feels so good not to be angry anymore."
Remorseful	"Oh, if only I could bring him back to his senses. I would tell him how much I loved him."
Resentful	"I only came to see you because my wife dragged me here."
Respectful	"You have a right to your feelings."
Sad	"My eyes are teary, and I feel like crying all the time."
Satisfied	"My children are good to me. They want me to have everything I need."
Shy	"I would like to tell you how I feel, but I never could express my feelings."
Spiritual	"Our beliefs help to create our experiences."
Tense	"I can't look you in the eye. When I talk to you I tap my fingers and get up and pace."
True Love	"I love you unconditionally."
Understood	"When I tell you about the difficulties I'm having, you seem to understand what I'm feeling."
Warm	"It was kind of you to share your good news with me."
Worthless	"I really don't matter to anyone—not even to myself."

PART TWO

Understanding and Dealing With the Patient's Problems

The good life is not a passive existence where you live and let live. It is one of involvement where you live and help live.
—ISAAC BASHEVIS SINGER

CHAPTER 10

The Physical Challenges of Alzheimer's Disease

Sometimes the patient with Alzheimer's disease forgets how to care for his own body. We learned how to dress ourselves and brush our teeth and eat our food so long ago that is seems as if we were born knowing how to do these things. Yet anyone who has toilet-trained a child, or watched him aim the spoon for his mouth and land it squarely on his ear, knows that all these behaviors, "activities of daily living," are learned. After they have been learned, they become autonomous—until physical damage to the brain causes the memory of that learned behavior to be partially or totally lost. If your loved one has lost some of these memories, you may find yourself once again patiently demonstrating the simplest tasks of everyday care. There may be moments when your sense of privacy, and your patient's, recoils at the necessity of helping him with bathroom habits and other personal tasks that we have been taught not to share. Yet, if we are aware of our own uncomfortable feelings and are able to discharge them or work them out, we can care for the physical aspects of a patient's needs in the same way we might care for a young and innocent child or a dear friend who is ill. In giving these needed physical services, we have the opportunity to show the patient with gestures and gentle words that he is loved and cared about.

Dressing and Grooming

Ms. Horvath: "I must set out my father's clean clothes, and take everything else away from him, or he will put his dirty clothes on again after he bathes."

Ms. Farmer: "My husband doesn't even seem to know what clothes to put on anymore. I've begun to set out for him, each morning, what he should wear. And still he gets mixed up. He doesn't know the difference between pajamas and underclothes or shirts. After he's all dressed in his undershirt and shorts, he'll come into the kitchen, and I'll see that he's put them on over his pajamas!"

Even people who have been very clothes-conscious all their lives can lose the ability to distinguish among different patterns or pieces of clothing. In the early stages of a memory-impairing illness, these patients can be helped by a rigorous labeling system. Dresser drawers are usually divided by type of clothing (shirts, underwear, socks, and so on) and can be labeled according to the contents. However, it can be more helpful to group all the items that are in one color family and that will go together even if they're not an exact match; for example, blue shirts, blue socks. When you buy new clothing for your relative, try to choose solid colors, which mix more readily than plaids and stripes.

Since your patient cannot necessarily tell you if he is too hot or too cold, you must be the judge and make sure he is dressed appropriately for the weather. Make your own adaptation, such as putting mittens on your relative instead of gloves. Mittens are warmer and easier to pull onto his hands.

Sometimes, labeling the drawers with pictures of clothing or providing simpler items of clothing is still not enough.

Mr. Castleton: "I'm right there, every morning. I've developed a certain routine. My brother no longer has any idea about what clothes to wear, so I set them out. Then I stay right with him until he's completely dressed. I don't simply leave things out for him because he isn't capable. He will put on the pajama pants again, unless I fold them and put them away the minute he takes them off. I can't leave him until he's dressed. Even then, I get frustrated. I'll hand his trousers to him, and he'll put his feet in them backwards. So I take them off and see that he gets them on right. Or he puts his shoes on the wrong feet. I must be there and supervise him completely.

"That's the way you cope. It lessens the tension on you, because you don't have to take things off and put them on again. And when he's all dressed, he'll stay that way. He won't undress."

SHAVING

Some men with Alzheimer's disease forget how to give themselves a shave. Since a man who is clean-shaven looks better and generally feels better than an unshaven one, caregivers should probably learn to shave their male patients. This activity may be difficult to adjust to by both caregiver and patient, but as Ms. Horvath's example demonstrates, inventiveness and a knowledge of her father's tastes and habits relieved her own embarrassment at her father's unshaven face and helped her father at the same time:

"I realized he wasn't shaving himself. And naturally, he didn't want me to do it for him. After all, I'm his daughter, and we hadn't lived together for thirty-five years. That's a very personal thing.

"So, when he first came to live with me, I took him to the barbershop, and when we got there I ordered a shave as well as a haircut for him, and then I told him that he couldn't have a haircut unless he got a shave."

Today he allows his daughter to shave him, and to prevent cutting herself or her father, Ms. Horvath uses an electric shaver. An old-fashioned ear syringe is used to blow the shavings out.

APPLYING MAKEUP

MR. ALTMAN: "My wife was always such a smart dresser; everything was always matched: her dress, her scarf, her shoes, her hair, and her makeup. I still try to keep her that way, even though she doesn't know how to dress herself anymore. Every Tuesday I take her to the hairdresser. He washes and sets her hair in a new style every week. He showed me how to brush her hair, and even though I was a little embarrassed, I asked him to teach me how to put some makeup on her— just a little color on her cheeks and some lipstick. I just can't get the hang of the eye makeup, but sometimes my daughter puts it on her.

"When we look in the mirror, she laughs, and I think she's pleased. She looks so pretty, and I tell her that. Then we go out to lunch like we used to. Sometimes it makes me forget just for a few minutes that she has problems with her memory and can't do anything for herself, or for me, anymore."

Assisting your relative with good grooming, and maintaining your own, will help both of you feel more attractive. Use the "act like" approach. When we "act like" we are more attractive, self-confident, or successful, we can feel that way.

PERSONAL HYGIENE

MR. WELDON: "My brother was a man who, before he got sick, wouldn't leave his house without showering. If there was something wrong with the water heater and the water was ice cold, he would take an ice cold shower. Now there are times when I can't get him into the shower. This morning, he finally agreed to take a shower. After his shower, I stayed right there to see that he dried, and that he got into his underwear. I supervised every minute."

MS. HORVATH: "My father has been a widower for twenty-five years. After my mother died, he lived alone and took care of himself. So, when he came to live with us, I figured he still would be able to care for himself. But soon after he arrived, we were invited to a family picnic, and I realized that he should have a shower or a bath before we went. When I suggested it, he refused and said he wouldn't do it. The smell . . . I was very embarrassed to take him anyplace."

When the smell of a dirty body belongs to a member of the family, someone you love and revere, your feeling of embarrassment is particularly heightened. Many caregivers have commented that they regarded their forgetful relative's inattention to cleanliness and grooming as a negative reflection on themselves. They fear that relatives and neighbors will think that they are not taking proper care of their forgetful loved ones. Then they blame themselves when they can't persuade their relative to observe good sanitary habits.

Many relatives have reported that their family members are "afraid" of the shower. We can only speculate on the reasons for their fearful reactions: perhaps they are afraid they will be hurt by the water, or they have forgotten how to adjust the temperature. Occasionally, victims of Alzheimer's disease suffer changes in their "internal thermostat" so that what may seem like a normal temperature to most of us will seem unbearably hot or cold to these patients. If you turn on the shower or bath, adjust the water temperature to make it tepid. As a safety precaution, set the water heater so that the water can never be scalding.

Bathing done at the same time each day or several times a week can become part of a regular routine that the impaired person comes to expect. Gradually, he will put up less resistance.

Bathing in a tub can be less threatening to the patient and easier for the caregiver to manage. Put nonslip grips or bathmats in the tub and run about three inches of water.

There remains the problem of physical size and strength, especially for the petite spouse or child dealing with a much larger person.

Ms. O'SHAUNESSY: "My husband's a big, tall man, six feet and 230 pounds. I can still manage him now, but I worry about what will happen when I can't physically handle him. I have to bathe him now, and so far our way of doing it is all right. He gets in the tub and sits, and he washes the front of his body. I keep a sharp eye on him, of course. I kneel down and wash his back and his head. Then I make him get out of the tub and dry himself because he can still do that himself."

Many caregivers have found that their patients will get in and out of the tub voluntarily if the persuasion is applied in a quiet, peaceful manner. Install grab bars so your patient can get in and out of the tub easily.

It's important not to get excited or nervous, or to threaten the person who objects to taking a bath. In some cases, you can administer a sponge bath while your relative is seated on a stool or on the toilet seat. Sometimes showering with the patient is the simplest solution.

Make sure he is thoroughly dried afterwards. To boost morale, use a refreshing after-bath scent and dry-skin lotion to keep the skin moisturized.

Often, caregiver children, siblings, and spouses are reluctant to deal with the personal hygiene of their relatives, especially where genital cleanliness is concerned. Because genitals are such private parts, relatives may object to being supervised while cleaning their genitals, or fight with someone who tries to do it for them.

Needless to say, it is extremely important that this area of the body be especially clean. Unwashed genitals produce an unpleasant smell and can harbor dangerous infections.

Two cousins lived together in a rather expensive apartment overlooking a lovely park. Marjorie Marble was 96, and Gladys Jamison ten years her junior. They were raised together just like sisters. Since their mothers had died early in life, the cousins combined their households. While the two depended on each other in many ways, it was Gladys, the younger, who took care of the home, even though she had studied to be a school teacher. Still physically able to care for herself at 86, despite some loss of hearing, Gladys also took care of her beloved first cousin.

Gladys was a good manager, but as she became a little feeble with age, her close friends insisted that she hire a homemaker to do the heavy household tasks—and especially to supervise Marjorie, who would sometimes become disoriented in the apartment and suspicious of

Gladys. The homemaker they hired, Ms. Molai, was a very pleasant, maternal, and understanding woman.

One day, while she was giving Marjorie her bath, Ms. Molai tried in a very casual but matter-of-fact way to wash Marjorie's genitals. Marjorie became enraged and started to scratch and bite Ms. Molai. It took what seemed like an eternity for Gladys and Ms. Molai to get her out of the bathtub. She continued to rant and rave for two more hours until, exhausted, she fell into a deep sleep.

When she awakened several hours later, Marjorie had forgotten the incident, but thereafter treated Ms. Molai with what appeared to be spiteful contempt. This incident in the bathtub apparently triggered a series of rages in Marjorie for which she eventually required medication.

Ms. Marble's reaction seemed directly related to the loss of her privacy and independence. Consider how you would feel in these circumstances, and use the same respectful gentleness that you would prefer to receive. Try to make bathing and toilet experiences as innocuous as possible. Remind your confused relative gently, or express tenderness and affection, just as you would to a child while performing a task that is distasteful to him.

ORAL HYGIENE

Oral hygiene is important, too. Ill-fitting dentures or mouth or gum infections can interfere with the Alzheimer's patient's ability to eat or chew the crunchy foods that provide needed roughage in the diet. Needless to say, an unwashed mouth has a terribly unpleasant odor. If your patient can brush his teeth under your supervision, of course, you can keep track of the health of his teeth and gums. If not, use the same approach as for bathing—quiet, calm persuasion: "I'm going to brush your teeth now. Open your mouth and look at me." Add a smile to make it easier. Dentures should be removed and cleaned daily, and the gums checked. For patients who object to the toothbrush, there are glycerine peroxide solutions that your dentist can recommend, or a pleasing flavorful mouthwash. Make sure these are not swallowed. Show your relative how to spit the liquid out.

Decreasing Physical Abilities
Add to Mental Confusion

As we grow older, all of us discover that while our body continues to be healthy, its strength and resilience have decreased. We need reading glasses, or a hearing aid, or sturdier, less fashionable shoes and are more likely to fall victim to some chronic conditions, such as diabetes, arthritis, or high blood pressure. Your elderly relative may also be suffering from reduced hearing or eyesight, or from some chronic physical problem, in addition to his forgetfulness and confusion. As a caregiver, you will want to monitor your memory-impaired relative's physical health, since illness and physical disability tend to increase mental confusion, while good physical health can significantly improve the patient's quality of life.

Lou Foster's mother had cataracts in her left eye for years. Because of her advanced age, the ophthalmologists said that since she could see out of her right eye they might as well leave well enough alone. Then she developed cataracts in the other eye. She became much more fearful of walking and was bumping into doors and walls. In fact, she was legally blind.

Finally, Lou found a doctor who was willing to undertake the surgery. At the age of 90, his mother had two intraocular transplants. Today, she sees, she walks around, she doesn't bruise herself, she can even read—although she doesn't remember what she's read.

It's hard to imagine the frustration she must have been feeling all that time, when not only could she not remember, she couldn't see! It was a very touching moment when the doctor took the bandage off and she looked at Lou, recognized his face, and smiled.

When your patient has defects in vision or hearing loss, these disabilities can cause difficulties not only with mobility, but also with communication, leading either to an inappropriate response or withdrawal into silence.

142

MEDICATIONS AND THEIR EFFECTS

As people grow older and are subject to more and more physical ailments, the number and kinds of medications they must take increase. Therefore, before your doctor prescribes any new drug for your relative, tell your doctor the current status of your patient's health, his medical history, any allergies to medications he may have, and all drugs he may be taking (including experimental drugs if he is part of a research program). Give the physician a complete description of the patient's symptoms.

Physicians, who often are unaware of the special requirements of the elderly patient with Alzheimer's disease, will occasionally prescribe medications that counteract a medication the patient is already taking, or perhaps prescribe too large a dose. It is always wise to ask your physician: "Will this medicine react with the tranquilizer (or insulin, or other drug) that he is already taking?" "What is the best time of day to give this medicine?" "What should I do if he misses a dose?" "Will smoking, drinking alcohol, or eating various foods interfere with the drug?" "On this drug, should he avoid the sun?" "Will this medicine make him drowsy?" "What are the possible side effects, and what should I do about them?" Don't assume that the doctor has consulted your patient's records or that he remembers every previous visit, treatment, or medication.

It is especially important to monitor the older person when he takes his medication. A memory-impaired person cannot be relied upon to medicate himself. Supervise him carefully to make sure that he doesn't overdose, but that he does swallow pills that are necessary for his well-being.

The side effects of medications may include drowsiness or its opposite, increased hyperactivity or agitation. Incontinence, rigidity of the muscles, a stooping and slow gait, falling, and peculiar movements of the hand or mouth are the side effects of several medications prescribed for the confused person. Sometimes tranquilizers meant to relax the patient have the opposite effect. In such a case a person who is given a tranquilizer may react, for instance, by throwing things and becoming hostile. If such an unexpected behavior should occur in the person for whom you are caring, alert your physician at once to these reactions and side effects. It may be necessary for the doctor to adjust the prescription by a process of trial-and-error until effective dosages of medication can be determined. In these situations, the caregiver is responsible for monitoring the patient's reactions, informing the physician, and in some cases deciding whether or not to continue a given drug.

Your pharmacist may be of utmost assistance in the matter of medication. He can catalog your patient's prescriptions. A pharmacist trained in geriatric pharmacology may be able to tell you which medications interact negatively with other drugs. Ask him to tell you which drugs should be listed on the patient's Medic Alert identification tags (see Chapter 12 for more information on Medic Alert).

How Much Do Physicians Really Know?

Perhaps we need to reexamine our traditional attitude toward the medical profession. Formerly, we put the physician on a pedestal. We saw him as an exceptional authority and expected him to know everything and to tell us how to run our lives. Today, we have to take more responsibility for our own care and the care of our chronically ill relatives.

Most general practitioners today are informing themselves about Alzheimer's disease and similar memory-impairing diseases. The best most of them can do, however, is to refer families to a neurologist or to a hospital with a research program. If the physician does not make such a referral, and you are not satisfied with his treatment, you may want to pursue more specialized help for your patient on your own. Your physician may not realize that your patient could benefit from the attention and experience of a neurologist or other specialist. All health-care professionals, including physicians, feel ignorant about these illnesses because there is so much that is not yet understood. What is very important is that there be one person who can direct you, the caregiver, in meeting the medical needs of your memory-impaired relative. That person may be a neurologist, family physician, psychologist, or internist, but it's very important to have one person who can examine your wife, husband, parent, or sibling, make a tentative diagnosis, and then suggest ways for you to proceed.

TREATING YOUR PATIENT'S PHYSICAL AILMENTS

Although Alzheimer's disease does not in itself generally cause pain, someone with this disease may be subject to the common cold, flu, virus, stomach cramps, sprained limbs, broken bones, cuts, bruises, sores, arthritis, rashes, sore gums, and so on. The symptoms of these illnesses may include fever, coughing, sneezing, vomiting, rapid pulse, diarrhea, flushing, difficulty in breathing, body swellings, dry skin, drowsiness, falling, convulsions, or hallucinations.

A sudden shift in behavior or refusal to do familiar things may be the only indication of an illness. All complaints about pain should be investigated. If you cannot find the cause of the pain, take your relative to a physician who will try to determine what is bothering him.

MRS. REICHOLD: "Last week my husband had a sore throat. At least, I think it was a sore throat, because he couldn't really tell me about it. All he could do was hold his throat and say, 'Me . . . me . . . me.' I took him to the doctor, but the doctor couldn't examine him because he refused to open his mouth. The doctor couldn't take his temperature or anything. My husband didn't get agitated and was very nice to the doctor and smiled at him, except whenever the doctor tried to do anything, he'd say, 'Not me, not me!' Finally, the doctor simply gave me a prescription for an antihistamine. That seemed to fix the problem, and it put him to sleep. He doesn't take any other medication, so I wasn't worried about the pills interacting with anything else."

MR. FORTH: "The night before last, my wife cut her right foot and, I think from where she was pointing, her heel. It was so painful that she couldn't step on it, and she'd lie on the bed with her foot off the edge. Now on the other leg she has an ulcerated ankle, but that didn't bother her. It doesn't hurt her or anything. I change the dressing three times a day.

"The next morning, I looked at her right foot, and there was nothing there! But she said it hurt, then it didn't, then it did . . . I didn't know whether it hurt or not. You don't know what to believe.

"Sometimes I think her feelings are different, or that she just can't tell me where it really hurts, although she can feel the pain."

It can become exasperating for a caregiver not to be able to assist the person who appears to be in pain. These situations tend to exaggerate our feelings of helplessness.

Yet, there are those moments, after one has been very worried about a husband or parent or wife, when the patient is healthy again and the situation is, in retrospect, even humorous.

Ms. Dignan: "My husband has a heart arrhythmia, and last winter the doctors decided that he ought to have a pacemaker implanted. I kept telling the doctors, 'Now, he doesn't understand you,' and they didn't believe me. Whenever they were talking to him, he would say his two words: 'You bet, you bet,' and they thought he was agreeing with them. Then, when they began to try to take some blood for tests, he changed to: 'You don't! You don't!' At one point during the examination, there were five people holding him down, and in spite of his heart problem, he still struggled away, saying, 'You don't! You don't!'

"Each one of those medical people thought that if they said to him, very quietly, 'We want to help you,' that when he said, 'You bet, you bet,' it meant he had understood. Then they would say, 'Now we are going to take some blood tests, is that all right?' And he would say, 'You bet, you bet.' Then they would begin and he would say, 'You don't, you don't!'

"Now, since they finally were able to install the pacemaker successfully, it's a funny picture to remember."

Eating

Eating is not, for most of us, simply a way to fuel and fortify our bodies; it is an act surrounded by memory and tradition and packed with emotional significance.

146

Beginning with our early experiences as suckling infants, food represents love and nurturance in our lives. As we grow older, we continue to focus on food and its meaning by shopping, cooking, and exchanging recipes; eating in restaurants; making party foods; becoming epicures or gourmands; or by overindulging in sweets, alcohol, and delicacies.

The older we get, the more important is the part that food plays in our lives. Perhaps paying attention to eating becomes our way of soothing the many losses and hurts that affect us as we age. Eating, at least, is one pleasure on which we can continue to depend. We fill up on food. Eating is a way to console ourselves; it makes us feel better. Thus, shopping for and preparing meals can become major activities in an older person's life.

At the same time, we are sometimes forced to accommodate our aging bodies by changing our eating habits. Difficulties with teeth and the need for partial or full dentures may be the first indications that lifelong food habits much change. This change can be the beginning of the decline of an older person's interest in food. Your elderly relative cannot chew the steak he used to enjoy; his teeth can't take the corn off the cob; his dentures trap raspberry seeds.

When your memory-impaired relative has difficulties with teeth and gums or wears dentures, you face the additional burden of providing him with a diet that is not only nourishing but tasty, chewable, and appealing as well.

Some caregivers have used baby foods as substitutes for hard-to-chew meat, vegetables, and fruits. Baby foods are uninteresting to the adult palate, but they are a way of obtaining a balanced and nutritious diet. Whole-grain bread and dairy products, such as cottage cheese and yogurt, can supplement and vary such fare.

When teeth or dentures are a problem, or when your relative has forgotten how to chew and swallow, or has developed other coordination problems, you must be alert to the possibility of his choking and try to prevent it.

Make sure foods are digestible and that the person chews his food well. Serve soft foods like those given to babies—applesauce, bananas, mashed potatoes, scrambled eggs, ground meat, and cottage cheese. Solid foods are best; combined liquids and solids—like cereal in milk—

may cause choking. Do not serve tough foods or crunchy snacks like hard candy or nuts, which need to be well chewed.

Learn the Heimlich maneuver, a technique to relieve a choking victim, so that, should your relative have an attack of choking, you will be able to help him. The Red Cross gives frequent classes to train people in this technique.

Elderly people sometimes experience reduced saliva production. Medication often causes drying of the mouth and decreases saliva. To compensate for this deficiency, serve moist food and liquids with each meal.

Some patients react to medications that dry the mouth (such as chlorpromazine and haloperidol) by producing excess saliva and drooling. (Various problems can make your patient drool, although reaction to medication is the most common; check with your physician as to the cause.)

In whatever form—water, juice, decaffeinated tea, or lukewarm soup—be sure your relative drinks enough fluids every day, especially during warm weather. It is vital that he does not become dehydrated. Fluids are necessary to avoid constipation and illness and to replace those lost from diarrhea or vomiting.

Dehydration may also occur in people who take water pills (diuretics) or heart medication or who have diabetes. Both thirst and unwillingness to drink can be symptoms of dehydration. Other possible signs are flushing and fever, rapid pulse, dizziness, and confusion. Sometimes, hallucinations result from severe dehydration. Ask your physician how much water your relative needs; each person requires an individual amount of liquids.

If the difficulties connected with eating exhaust your patient rather quickly, don't force him to eat a large meal all at once. Serve smaller portions more frequently (eating five or six small meals is healthier than eating three large ones).

Whatever form your relative's diet may take, you will want to try to prevent nutritional deficiencies in the diet of a memory-impaired elderly person so that you can expect him to continue to be physically healthy and as productive as his capabilities allow.

Deficiencies in nutrition have been implicated in chronic constipation, fragile bones and bone loss (as in osteoporosis), diabetes, high blood pressure, heart disease, stroke, and cancer. In addition, poor nutrition aggravates mental problems.

Some individuals are diagnosed as being senile and put into nursing homes because they appear to be disoriented and confused, have severe memory lapses, and seem delusional. They may actually be suffering from malnutrition and anemia. In many of these cases, when the elderly person is diagnosed quickly enough and treated early and appropriately with nutritious meals and tender loving care, the "senility" appears to be reversible and the individual is able to return to independent functioning that is appropriate for his age.

The problems with eating, drinking, chewing, and swallowing associated with Alzheimer's and similar diseases can make mealtimes very difficult for your relative—and very trying for you. Yet, as many caregivers have learned from experience, if your relative senses your exasperation or feels hurried or pressured, his agitation and his eating problems are likely to increase. To avoid major problems, try to stick to a constant mealtime routine, serving the patient at regular hours each day and in the customary way each time. Maintain as calm and pleasant an atmosphere as possible.

When people are upset they may eat too much or have no appetite at all because our emotions affect our appetite. If mealtimes are unpleasant, hurried times, then the impaired person may either not eat at all or demand more food as a way of getting your solicitude.

Serve soup in a cup; it's easier than handling a bowl and a spoon. For patients with more advanced impairment, use your ingenuity to make adaptations such as Mr. Tate's:

> "I've learned to cook since my wife became ill—nothing fancy, but it serves. However, I also work full-time, so I must prepare our meals ahead of time and freeze them so they can simply be warmed up at dinnertime.
>
> "Now I have an additional problem. My wife no longer wants to eat off a plate. She wants a small plate, or better yet, a bowl. I bought some oven-proof casserole dishes, and I make up the meals, such as a stew or

casserole and meatballs, right in the dishes. They're appetizing-looking, and she doesn't object to eating from the casserole."

If your relative has forgotten how to feed himself, or is having trouble coordinating his actions, try "patterning": take the spoon and place food on it; then put the spoon in the patient's hand. Gently assist him to guide the spoon into his mouth. Remind him to chew and swallow (to forestall choking). Repeat this process and at the same time praise your relative's ability to feed himself independently. You are using a conditioning technique that can be useful to you with other problem behaviors as well as with eating.

Add milk and sugar to tea and coffee before you serve it, and make sure it is warm, not hot, to avoid burning your relative's mouth to tongue. Memory-impaired patients appear to lose their sense of hot and cold and may burn their mouths on hot foods.

Many choices of food on a plate confuse an impaired person. Serve one part of the meal at a time. Plan simple menus, featuring one-dish meals, as Mr. Tate did. Keep the number of forks, spoons, and knives to a minimum—sometimes one spoon is sufficient, and the lack of choice discourages playing with the silverware.

Serve sandwiches that are already cut up in quarters so your relative won't need to use a knife. Other foods that can be eaten with the fingers are raw fruits and vegetables cut into slices, which are easier to handle, and deboned chicken legs or thighs.

Don't keep condiments, such as sugar, salt, spices, ketchup, oil, or vinegar, within easy reach or you may find all of them dumped in your relative's plate. Similarly, the dog's biscuits, artificial flowers or fruit, or anything colorful that looks like food may also become the meal of the day. Don't keep them around.

Also, don't insist that a person eat if he is sleepy or irritable. Missing one meal is not a calamity; insisting that a person eat may cause one.

Every family member, including the memory-impaired person, should have his own place at the table.

If your patient wants to help in mealtime preparation, give him a small job to do: peeling carrots or potatoes, cutting fruit, setting the table (wrap the silverware in a napkin so he won't be confused about where each utensil should be placed). He may be able to wash or dry the dishes. It will give your relative a sense of purpose to contribute his labor.

While mealtime is often a problem for the caregiver, it can be a good time to disguise medication so that your patient will swallow it and not spit it out, hold it under his tongue, give it to the dog, or drop it in the fishbowl.

> Ms. Cooper: "My brother has forgotten how to swallow pills, but he must take his high-blood pressure medicine every day. So I crush his pill and put it in applesauce. You could use scrambled eggs, if they're soft, or oatmeal, or any food with a strong flavor and a creamy consistency. I coat the spoon with it and he takes it right from me. It's a technique I learned when my children were small."

Giving medication is a vitally important part of caring for an elderly person with some memory loss. Frequently, the elderly patient has other problems that may or may not be associated with his memory impairment. As we age, some of our body's organs weaken or become diseased. Your relative may be taking a tranquilizer to reduce agitation, insulin for a diabetic condition, digitalis or other heart medication, and vitamins, sleeping pills, or diuretics as well. Each of these medications has its own schedule, its own requirements for administration (with food, without food, before bedtime, and so on), and its own side effects.

BEHAVIORS THAT DISRUPT MEALTIMES

Many families find that their forgetful relative develops behaviors that disrupt normal mealtime activities. These behaviors may be due to physical disabilities, loss of memory of eating skills and table manners, or decreased coordination. Whatever the cause, your impaired family member will benefit from your inventiveness and consideration in adapting to his new needs. Like you, other families have faced the problems that mealtimes present and have tried to create their own solutions. Some of their experiences may help you.

MR. BOEHM: "My wife was going to the senior citizen's center every day because I was working full-time and couldn't leave her at home alone. They serve a terrific hot lunch at the center. But last December the director called me up and said, 'Your wife cannot eat on her own anymore. If you don't come and feed her, we can't have her here, because she disrupts everybody.' Her hands were going all over the place, like a baby's hands. They had tried other solutions—some of the other senior citizens who are volunteers had tried to feed her, but she wouldn't cooperate.

"So I spoke to my boss, who agreed to put me on half-days. Now I drive my wife to the center in the morning, then come back at lunchtime to feed her."

MR. COBBLER: "My wife and I used to go out for dinner fairly often. Now it's very difficult to take her out because her eyesight has become quite poor and you can't find a brightly lit restaurant. They're all fairly dark in the evening, and she can't find her way in and out, or see what she's eating, or read the menu. The whole situation makes her really unhappy, and she wants to go home. So we don't eat out as often as we used to. That's the only way I can handle it. I keep telling my friends: 'If you know of brightly lit restaurant nearby, don't keep it a secret, OK?' "

MR. FRANTZ: "My wife seems to have an insatiable hunger. She has absolutely no memory of having eaten a meal. Ten minutes later she'll say, 'I'm starved. I want something to eat.' Or else she'll say, 'Did I already eat?' or, 'Is it time to eat?' right after I've cleared the table.

"I can't tell whether she's asking to eat because she enjoys eating, or whether she's bored and wants something to do, or whether she simply doesn't remember what she did ten minutes ago. It would seem to me that if she had just eaten a meal she should feel full, and notice the feeling. But that doesn't seem to matter.

"She expects me to prepare something, so there are times when I think it's the attention she craves. I generally offer her an apple or a piece of fruit, which won't put weight on her, and try to divert her attention.

Sometimes I'll say, 'We'll eat in a little while, after we finish what we're doing.' She doesn't really need to eat again!"

The desire to eat right after the meal is over stems from a lack of memory of the experience of having eaten. Eating is such a very important experience to all of us that it has a great deal of emotional significance and carries complex meanings.

There also can be a great deal of frustration and conflict over the eating experience. (You know how many wrangles you may have had with your children over food when, for example, they wanted to eat and you said they had to wait.) For adults, food and mealtimes are still invested with positive and negative feelings, but unfortunately, we don't know what the feelings are that a confused or memory-impaired person may be experiencing. It may be that he's not eating enough at the meal; but if he can be sated by fruit or a snack of carrots, celery, or cheese and crackers, then you know that his need is not physiological, that he's not demanding food because he is actually hungry. Perhaps, like Mrs. Frantz, he wants more attention from you. In any case, the forgetful person's frequent desire to eat can have unhealthy consequences for his weight.

Ms. KOLODNY: "My uncle is in very good health. Unfortunately, he has begun to put on weight. He always had a good appetite. Now, he seems positively ravenous. He'll reach across and take food off my plate when he's finished his own.

"He used to be quite a snacker, too. He was always going into the refrigerator or into the cupboard or the pantry for a nibble. Now he never looks in the cupboards or the refrigerator—I think he's forgotten that food is in there. He does go into the candy jar that is sitting on the end table in the library. I've put low-calorie candies in that, so eating out of it won't put too much weight on him."

On the other hand, some memory-impaired people forget to eat at all:

Ms. NORBETT: "About a year ago, my husband stopped eating. He refused to have any food. That was a problem. The doctor gave me a liquid that I fed him for about three months. Then he went back to taking solid food, if I would feed him. He has to be fed like a baby of six months. He eats slowly. Sometimes he's not able to control his chewing and his swallowing. We have to give him soft foods that are easy to chew."

If they stop eating, or especially if they become dehydrated, memory-impaired patients may develop viral or bacterial pneumonia, of which the first sign may be delirium. Memory loss often worsens when they become ill.

Because patients with Alzheimer's disease frequently die of pneumonia, the caregiver should be on the alert for any signs of refusal to eat solid foods. Patients who stop eating can be fed a liquid diet that will help to keep up their strength. If your relative develops pneumonia, either at home or in a nursing home, he should have immediate medical attention.

An impaired person may have forgotten the concept of "food" and may eat things that look like food. Mrs. Constanza speaks of her husband:

"He's lost the concept of food, unless it's right there in front of him. If I don't have his plate set right on the table with the food in it, he won't know what to eat. For instance, if I have a bouquet of flowers on the table when he sits down, but his plate isn't there yet, he'll eat the flowers."

Forgetting Good Toilet Habits

The same recent memory that reminds us when we ate our last meal also reminds us how recently we urinated or had a bowel movement. The forgetful older person may not remember how long it has been since he went to the bathroom. He may also not remember how to respond to the warning signals his body sends him; a full feeling in his bladder or bowel will not connect in his mind with the need to do something about it. As a result, he may have an "accident," which can be an excruciatingly embarrassing experience for him (if he's aware that he's wet) and for you.

Toilet behavior is a very private behavior for most people. Bringing this intimate aspect of a relative's life to his attention may be extremely embarrassing for both him and his family. In addition, your intrusion into what he perceives as his privacy may threaten him and increase his agitation.

While you cannot ignore your relative's problems with toilet habits— for he may well need your help—it is very important in this area of daily life to express tenderness and affection while performing anything that may be distasteful to you both. In that way you can be most helpful and comforting to your forgetful spouse, sibling, or parent.

There will probably be a certain amount of awkwardness when you first attempt to take charge of your patient's toilet habits. Since when we are embarrassed we are more likely to become irritated or angry, it is especially important to manage our own feelings while helping our impaired relative. Try to be calm, reassuring, unhurried, specific, and matter-of-fact as you take your relative to the bathroom, undress him, and encourage him to urinate or defecate.

Many caregivers have succeeded in coping with their forgetful patients' toilet problems. Some of their suggestions and solutions may help you.

> MR. HEALY: "I have to remind my wife, every two hours, that she has to go to the bathroom. That's during the day. At night, even after taking a sleeping pill, she'll get up to go to the bathroom. I try not to let her have anything to drink after eight o'clock. I leave a night-light on—one in the hall and one in the bathroom. Even so, last night she urinated all over the toilet seat. She was half asleep; she didn't know. I told her to lift up the cover, but it was too late. I should remember to leave the cover up when I go to bed, like my son suggested."

Put a picture and sign over the toilet that show how to "Wipe Yourself" and "Flush" to remind the memory-impaired person about what he should do after going to the toilet. A sign saying "Wash Your Hands," or a picture over the sink showing someone washing his hands, can also be a helpful hint.

For safety and convenience, install grab bars that the Alzheimer's patient can grasp to lift himself off the toilet. A raised and padded toilet seat makes sitting a long time more comfortable and affords easier access to the toilet from a wheelchair. If the bathroom is upstairs and the bedroom downstairs, you may decide to install a portable commode next to the patient's bed to spare him the frantic rush to the toilet and the possibility of accidents during the climb upstairs. These items are obtainable, for purchase or rent, from a local medical supply house. Medicare and Medicaid cover some or all of the cost of renting them if a physician orders their use.

Sometimes the Alzheimer's patient may become confused when he is taken to the bathroom—after a meal, for instance—and he doesn't know what is expected of him:

> Ms. Patricks: "The other day, when my teenage daughter took my sister to the bathroom, Mary (my sister) got completely undressed instead of just sitting on the toilet. While my daughter was waiting outside the door, Mary took off her dress, underwear, shoes, and socks—and then I had to completely redress her. My daughter had neglected to sit Mary down and instruct her. It was my fault, though, because I should have told her how to handle it—she was only trying to be helpful."

It is very important that whoever assists in caregiving, including young or teenage children (who can be very helpful), be given explicit instruction about the patient's condition and how to handle it. In Ms. Patrick's case, no real harm was done, but her daughter was baffled by her aunt's confused behavior because she didn't expect it.

A son may be embarrassed to take his mother to the toilet, especially to a public rest room.

When Mr. Braun and his mother are out in public, such as in a department store or a hotel, he has a mental ready-reference list of ladies' rooms that have attendants. His mother is not incontinent, but she has no way of gauging herself, so he tries to get her to the ladies' room frequently. He slips up to the door, signals to the attendant, and explains to her that his mother will get lost. If the attendant is willing to take care of her, he usually tries to tip her, although some of the attendants refuse.

The smell of urine that drips onto panties and other clothing leaves an unpleasant odor of which the Alzheimer's victim is not aware. But relatives cringe when they realize what has caused it.

Mrs. Ackerman lived in a downstairs apartment in her son's house. Every day she cooked for herself, cleaned her apartment, got neatly dressed, and then went to the senior citizens' center two blocks away. Harold Ackerman and his wife realized that his mother was sometimes confused and forgetful, but since she could manage independently, they felt she should continue to live in her apartment by herself.

One day Janet Ackerman got a phone call from the senior center, asking that Mrs. Ackerman not return to the center because other members in the center could not tolerate her smell. Janet and Harold felt terribly embarrassed and discussed the matter with his mother, who denied that she knew what they were talking about.

It was then that Janet and Harold decided that Mrs. Ackerman could no longer live alone. Although her ability to function appeared intact, she had been neglecting to bathe and wore the same soiled underwear, which smelled of feces. She continually soiled herself and did nothing about it. Her son and daughter-in-law were not aware of her incontinence until it was brought to their attention by the social worker at the senior citizen's center.

Some relatives, such as Mr. Brummage, have found in themselves the inner reserves to go beyond embarrassment when faced with the confused behavior of their impaired family member:

"I like to take my father to the baseball game, even though I'm not sure he knows what's going on in the game. The atmosphere in the park is something he is comfortable with, because he's known it all his life. I always have to make sure he goes to the men's room. He's not incontinent, but he doesn't always give himself enough time to get to a bathroom, so I always take him to the men's room first.

157

"They have a new kind of urinal that looks like a washbasin. Last time I took him there, he stood in front of it, and he knew I wanted him to do something, but he had no idea what. Finally he reached his hands down and washed them in the urinal. Of course, everybody stood around staring at him, and at me.

"But, at this point, I have gone way beyond embarrassment. I found it didn't trouble me at all, although it would have a couple of years ago."

CONSTIPATION AND DIARRHEA

The person whose memory is impaired, unfortunately, cannot always keep track of his bowel movements. Because of lack of exercise, the effect of medications, the slowing of digestion, or improper diet, including too much refined sugar and not enough fiber or roughage, the Alzheimer's patient may become constipated. Usually the first symptoms of constipation are abdominal pain and a headache.

While it is unpleasant to have to keep track of your relative's bowel habits, and although the person may feel intruded upon, it is essential that you do so. Be as discreet as possible so that neither of you becomes too embarrassed. Constipation can be very painful and add to the confusion of the patient. If his bowel is blocked or impacted, and the body can therefore not rid itself of its waste products, consult a nurse or physician.

Diets rich in fiber include whole-grain foods such as whole-wheat bread, bran muffins or cereal, brown rice, and wheat germ. Stewed or fresh fruits and green leafy vegetables also add dietary fiber. Foods rich in vitamin B, such as whole-grain cereals and breads, help in preserving muscle tone in the digestive tract. Nuts, raw vegetables, and granola, if your relative can still chew and swallow easily, are high in fiber and make tasty snacks.

Fluid intake should equal at least eight glasses of water or juices per day. Prune juice or warm water with lemon decreases constipation. Don't administer laxatives unless they are prescribed by the physician. When in doubt, ask.

Daily exercise, such as a long walk, will help your confused relative to have more regular bowel movements. While each of us has a bowel movement at different intervals, it is normal to have one at least every second or third day.

As with constipation, diarrhea may also be caused by the patient's inadequate eating habits. However, diarrhea may also be a symptom of influenza or food poisoning, or may be due to medications or emotional upset.

Treat the diarrhea symptomatically. Give your relative clear liquids such as bouillon or clear broth, ginger ale, weak sweetened tea, and juices. Gradually add solid foods that are rich in carbohydrates. Foods that are binding include gelatin desserts, bananas, and toast (unbuttered). Avoid butter and other foods high in fat; avoid vegetables, fruits, whole grains, and meats until the diarrhea subsides. Then resume a nutritious diet.

INCONTINENCE

The inability to control one's need to eliminate urine or feces is known as incontinence. It may be caused by central nervous system damage or by the loss of control of sphincter muscles that enable us to hold the urethra and anus closed. Sometimes incontinence is caused by stress, as when we are excited, frightened, tearful, or laughing hysterically. Certain medications and infections also account for some incontinence.

In the early stages of a memory-impairing disease, most incontinence is urinary. The first possible cause to consider is diet—is your relative taking in large quantities of liquid at any specific time? By observing the patterns of liquid intake and incontinence, you can put your memory-impaired patient on a bladder-emptying schedule: every two or three hours, before and after meals, and just before bedtime.

Bladder training, with exercises to tighten the muscle tissue by interrupting the flow of urine in midstream, is useful if your relative can comprehend your requests. In nursing homes, bladder and bowel training can be successful in the early stages, unless Alzheimer's disease causes uninhibited neurogenic bladder. Regaining control over these functions can restore one's dignity and self-esteem.

If the patient leaks urine, sometimes the use of diapers or sanitary napkins can alleviate some of the smelly discomfort. Use deodorants around your house, and on the impaired relative when possible, to dissipate any odors.

MS. VALENTE: "I use what they call 'adult briefs,' which are like diapers, for my sister. During the day she's hardly ever incontinent, so this is merely a safeguard, just in case I don't get her to the bathroom in time. With the briefs, she won't be wet or chafed, and she won't wet the bed at night. They are basically diaperlike, adjustable rubber pants into which you insert an absorbent pad. If the briefs won't stay in place by themselves, you can put underpants over them.

"Although you are probably supposed to put them on while she is lying down, I can't do that because she's too heavy, so my sister stands up and holds on to the grab bar in the bathroom while I put them on and insert the pad from behind. Perhaps, too, it's a little less embarrassing that way—she doesn't have to watch me. I admit it took me a long time to do it without feeling upset about it. You don't have the same feeling as you would diapering a baby."

When incontinence comes and goes, the problem may be psychological in origin. Patients who are angry or disappointed sometimes show how they feel by urinating or defecating on the floor. If you suspect this is what is going on, try to find out what's bothering your relative. He may not be able to tell you outright, but by being sensitive to him, you may be able to discover the underlying cause and correct the situation. Then the incontinence symptom will disappear either for good or until the next time he is upset.

No matter how upsetting (or trivial) the problem may seem, discuss all incidents of incontinence with your doctor, who may be able to help you. Mrs. Drake was having an occasional problem with incontinence. Their doctor suggested to Mr. Drake that he provide his wife with a catheter attached to a bag—the type used in the hospital after an operation. Since the administration of a catheter requires the cooperation of the patient, Mr. Drake worried that it may not be so simple for a nonprofessional to accomplish; Mrs. Drake wasn't usually all that accommodating. Later, if her accidents get to be more frequent, a catheter might be a viable solution.

If you know when your relative usually has a bowel movement, you can take him to the toilet before that time and avoid accidents. Stool softeners, available at the drugstore, are helpful to ease bowel movements. A comfortable bathroom with bar supports to hold on to will encourage your relative to sit long enough to defecate. Giving him a magazine to glance at and music to listen to may help to create a comfortable atmosphere.

When you can't get your relative to the bathroom on time, don't blame yourself. Accidents do happen, and you're only human.

Use disposable pads, rubber sheets, or plastic pads in between sheets to protect your bedding and keep it clean and dry.

> Ms. WYLYS: "I use a waterproof mattress pad made of reversible vinyl-coated polyester. I put absorbent pads on top of that and then the sheet. The mattress pad is washable, even though it's waterproof, so it can be put in the machine. It's also odorproof, but from time to time it should be sprayed with a disinfectant. Many major department stores carry them in their linen departments, but you have to ask. Be prepared for people to say, 'We don't carry it,' although they usually have it hidden away on a shelf."

If there are accidents, it is best not to fuss about them. Clean the person up and try to manage your feelings while doing so. Try to resist the temptation to take out your frustration on the patient. Go back to some of our suggestions for managing your anger and handling stress. They will help you at this critical time.

Make your relative's toilet pattern as simple and bearable a part of your daily life as possible. Use the tension relievers that we have suggested to help you. When fecal incontinence occurs, it is often "the last straw" for many relatives because it is so distressing and unpleasant. Its advent motivates some caregivers to make the decision to place their impaired relative in a nursing home, suggesting the difficulties of dealing with the many and varied problems of the victims of Alzheimer's disease.

Exercise and Recreation for the Patient

All of us need good nutrition and a certain amount of exercise to function well, including our impaired relatives. Because they have no memory of and cannot motivate themselves to exercise, even if they were athletic in the past, the caregivers must direct the activity.

Walking is an excellent form of exercise that is available to most of us. Many caregivers make it a habit to take a long walk with their confused patient every day. They travel the same route, reminding the forgetful person of familiar sights and acquaintances they meet. One man takes his brother to lunch at the same restaurant every day. Not only does the trip relieve him of the necessity of cooking, but also the walk is good exercise, and both he and his brother enjoy the opportunity to get out, stretch, and take a break from the house and its routine.

If the weather is bad and there isn't too much space in your house or apartment, practice walking in rhythm, and time yourself. Walking briskly, as if to a marching tune (and even better, with music playing in the background to keep time to), may be an enjoyable activity for both of you. Who said exercise can't be fun?

Calisthenics can be adjusted to any skill level, done in or out of doors, performed with a partner, in a group, or by yourself. When you exercise, do a specific exercise first, and then ask your patient to do the same. If necessary, gently guide him with your hands, but don't force the issue.

If your relative has arthritis or some other medical condition that makes movement a problem, ask a physical therapist to recommend special exercises for him.

For recreation, draw on past activities of the patient if he is still able to do the activity and seems to enjoy it. Caregivers have reported that their impaired relatives continue to play tennis and golf even as they are becoming more severely impaired and less able to do things for themselves. It seems that lifelong habits and pursuits that were extremely enjoyable persist the longest, even in a patient with substantial memory loss. Playing the piano is another skill that may remain, and one that may delight the impaired person. He may enjoy singing or hearing familiar music on records, on the radio, or in a concert hall.

Some memory-impaired patients, even though they are incapable of following the plot of a story, may enjoy watching television. Others, however, develop delusions and become paranoid; they think that the people on the television are talking about them, or plotting against them.

MR. ROSS: "Do you know how I survived the winter? 'I Love Lucy' at 7:30 every night. A laugh a night—you have to have a laugh. My wife always watches it with me. She enjoys it. The slapstick she can understand, but anything else. . . . And sometimes I'd find a movie for us to go see. Anything sad would make her fidgety, so I would find the funniest movies I could.

"At the end of the winter, I was practically stir-crazy. I was like a nut by nightfall. We couldn't go out for a walk at night yet; it was dark too early, and still too cold. I'd go through the television listings to find something funny—a laugh a night."

Dancing is an activity that many couples have developed as a lifelong recreational pursuit. Even when one member of the couple has lost some of his memory, he may still remember all the steps to the dances and enjoy the music and the social occasion. The partner whose memory is intact must be aware, though, that people may notice some peculiar behaviors of the spouse. Be prepared for some questions or comments if your partner forgets who the other dancers are or can't find the way to the rest room. You can explain honestly to your fellow dancers that, at times, your spouse experiences memory losses.

Is your relative still able to read? Perhaps Mr. Lorenzo's experience will help you. Mr. Lorenzo thought his wife had completely lost the ability to read, and that was a terribly sad event because she had been a writer and a book reviewer and reading was extremely important to her. She would get bored with the newspaper and magazines, so he bought a book of short stories in large type. She can read now for an hour at a time, because they're short stories, and they're funny and she can grasp them. The newspaper had very poor print, and the stories were long. She probably had difficulty understanding the material in the complex political and economic stories.

TAKE ADVANTAGE OF PREVIOUS SKILLS AND KNOWLEDGE

Jeremy Jordan was an architect of children's playgrounds and pediatric facilities and, in his spare time, a wonderful painter of children's portraits. When Jeremy became ill, his wife Sheila tried to encourage him to continue painting. But he put away his oils, brushes, and canvases. Sometimes, to coax Jeremy into painting again, Sheila would take out his sketchbook and show him photographs of his paintings. He would stare at the pictures and smile; but he refused to take up a brush or to touch his sketchbook and charcoal. Somehow he knew he could no longer capture on canvas the complexities of a child's face.

Jeremy was merely 52 when he developed Alzheimer's disease. Sheila wept for his lost abilities every time she thought of the wasted years to come, years in which his talent might otherwise have continued to flourish.

Desperate to find a meaningful activity for Jeremy, Sheila got him to begin to use his senses again. She brought flowers into the house and showed him how to smell, touch, and even taste the roses and the cherry blossoms. When Jeremy seemed to enjoy this, she took him out into the woods with her where he helped her gather berries for jam. By helping Sheila and participating in her hobby, Jeremy gained both stimulation and companionship. No longer need he spend hours alone in the house.

Diversion from one activity to another is usually more relaxing even for the memory-impaired person that complete rest. Total inactivity is frustrating. Meaningless activity, in which there is no sense of usefulness or challenge, is deadening even for the person who has lost his memory.

While victims of Alzheimer's disease and other similar diseases may have a reduced capacity for intellectual activity, that capacity is not completely eliminated. They can respond to activity at some level. It may be more difficult for you to devise ways to entertain your impaired relative, but the rewards can be substantial, both for him and for you. Going out can be a relief for you as well as for your spouse or parent. Many memory-impaired people have lost the ability to amuse themselves, because self-enjoyment generally involves memory over an extended period—a memory capacity that they no longer possess. However, they have not lost all of the ability to be amused or to feel good.

The forgetful person may not be able to tell you what he likes, but he can respond to your stimulation, whether you present him with something pretty to see, to hear, to taste, to smell, or to touch. Touch may be the only remaining communicative bond between you. A gentle touch, a caress, a kiss, holding hands—all communicate tenderness and love. And when you give love, it is bound to return to you, whether in a word, a glance, or a smile.

MRS. VORHEES: "One of the things that my husband could always do is play poker. He still plays poker with friends one night a week. And his poker is just as good as it was; he was a fairly good player. There doesn't seem to be any deterioration. He remembers the winning sequences and the betting; it amazes me. I don't understand it. In other respects, his memory is not good. He's forever misplacing things in the house."

MR. CANCORT: "There's one thing my wife can still do, and that is play cards. I don't know how to figure it out. She can play bridge, but she remembers nothing else—names, addresses, yesterday's paper—but she knows the cards that are out. I have a good memory and I don't know bridge as well as she does. To me, it's very strange."

We are often perplexed when we hear that a person with a memory-impairing disease is still able to dance, or to play cards, chess, tennis, or golf. Usually these abilities and skills are present during the early stages of the illness; however, sometimes people who have been afflicted for four or five years are still capable of these activities. When these abilities remain they are sustaining to the individual.

If your relative retains such an ability, provide opportunities to continue these activities as long as possible. They are probably a source of pleasure and comfort for him, and we can speculate that, in some way, they may even delay further deterioration.

CHAPTER 11

The Psychological Toll of Memory Loss

*A*lzheimer's disease and similar memory-impairing illnesses usually develop very slowly. For this reason, a person who is in the beginning stages of such a disease may be aware, from time to time, that there is something wrong with his memory. This is such an extremely difficult discovery to accept that some people deny that anything is amiss. They project their forgetfulness and communication problems onto others. Thus, they may blame the caregiver for hiding things or failing to tell them about important decisions or events. Accusations are insulting and painful for the caregiver. They emanate from the humiliation your relative may feel when he forgets something important; the realization that his memory is slipping away may just be too frightening.

Some people who develop memory impairment are both intellectually and emotionally aware that their mental processes are not working as well as before. That recognition, in the early stages of the illness, may cause psychological difficulties over and above the memory loss. Your relative may become embarrassed, frustrated, angry, or depressed about the implications of his condition.

At this point, the Alzheimer's patient can benefit from psychotherapy. He will learn through psychotherapy to accept and deal with his disability, as well as some techniques for living with an imperfect memory and ways of compensating for it. Memory enhancement programs teach the patient how to cope with everyday situations more effectively. One method is for the patient to train himself to actively look, listen, and talk about an action as it occurs, thus enhancing his memory of it. For example, as he takes off his glasses, he says to himself, "I'm putting my glasses on the desk." When he goes into the kitchen, he can state, "I'm going to turn on the gas under the coffee." These actions make it more likely that he will remember where he put down his glasses and that water is boiling in the next room.

Patients can also learn to control their physical environment. If, for instance, a patient wishes to take some clothes to the laundry, putting the laundry bag in front of the door is a good way not to forget. Family members can help the patient by setting up a highly structured environment:

- Label drawers, cabinets, and closets with pictures and words.
- Post a list of important names and numbers by all phones.
- Put up signs showing where important rooms or items are located.

The benefit of openly discussing the illness with the patient is that it prepares him for the changes he will undergo, while allowing him to get his affairs in order, such as appointing a guardian to manage financial affairs and allowing him to make decisions about how he wants to spend his remaining time. Decision-making will be much easier once the Alzheimer's patient recognizes that telling family members about the illness and planning for the future—including getting help in the house—can be accomplished in the very early stages before lapses in memory and coherence become more serious and longer lasting.

When Mrs. Baker was diagnosed as having Alzheimer's, she was aware of the deterioration she would undergo, as she had seen both her father and grandfather suffer the effects of the disease. Her husband decided that he would retire from his job to devote his time to helping her do the things that made her feel comfortable. She wanted to continue to live as before, at home, doing her housekeeping chores as best she could. Each month they traveled to see one of their six children and spent a week visiting, talking about Mrs. Baker's feelings about herself, her illness, her hopes and dreams for the future of her children and grandchildren, including specifics, such as when she would really need to be confined, where and how she wanted this to occur, what she wanted her children to have, and her husband's future life. A woman of great courage, she made a television appearance to let people know her thoughts and feelings and to encourage them not to be afraid of the disease and its victims.

Perhaps Mrs. Baker's practical and energetic mental outlook enabled her to be lucid for longer than anticipated. While this is speculative, we do know that a strong will can sometimes affect the course of an illness.

On the other hand, a patient may go into inexplicable rages, become suspicious, or have hallucinations or delusions. It is helpful to understand these reactions and what you can do about them.

MR. CORWIN: "From what we've been able to learn, my mother has a 'classic case' of Alzheimer's disease. She is still well enough to understand the problem, and to tell us her feelings.

"Her biggest problem is the fact that she knows she's sick. She's very embarrassed by what she calls the weakness of her mind. She needs a therapy group or some counseling as much as I do. I'm surprised there isn't something for her.

"When she first became ill, she thought she was losing her mind, and the first thing we did was to send her to a psychologist. She was very pleased to find out she has a disease and that she isn't 'crazy.' But I think she's insulted by what is happening to her; sometimes she seems foolish in the way she tries to compensate. She knows, when she talks, that it isn't coming out right. And she'll say the same thing two or three times, but sometimes I can't understand what she's trying to say. Then she seems embarrassed.

"Her shame about having this illness seems to be harming her as much as the illness itself."

Verbal Communication with Your Memory-Impaired Relative

MS. BETTY PFALZ: "There seems to be a problem that many people with memory problems have in using the right word for the right item. Take my brother, who doesn't call a handkerchief a 'handkerchief' anymore. He calls it a 'napkin.' My friend Marie's husband calls it a 'sword,' of all things. And Mr. Eden from the support group says his wife calls it an 'apron.' "

While we don't know precisely what causes this confusion in a person with Alzheimer's disease, it can be compared to a short circuit in the central switchboard of a telephone system. Each time you pick up your telephone and dial a next-door neighbor, the call is switched across town. The memory-impaired person, seeing a glass of water on the table and wanting a drink, may have lost the word for drink or water. He might call the water glass a "plate," or ask for a "think," for example, confusing either category or sound, because the connections between image and word have been scrambled.

Both Thomas Newington and his daughter Sandra were lawyers. When Mr. Newington developed Alzheimer's disease in his late sixties, Sandra was already living and practicing law in another city, but they kept in frequent touch by phone. "For a person who was as literate and verbal as my father had always been, not being able to find the right word was frustrating, and he would become extremely angry as a result," Sandra recalls. "One day when I was chatting with Dad, we got onto the subject of breakfast, and suddenly he said, 'You could have a peanut for breakfast.'

" 'A peanut?' I said. 'Daddy, why would I want a peanut for breakfast?'

" 'Because then you could trade it for one of those round yellow things.'

" 'Do you mean an egg?' I asked him. 'Or a lemon?'

" 'No, no,' he said, 'the big yellow round thing.'

" 'A grapefruit?' I asked.

" 'Yes, that's what I mean.' "

While it took some patience on Ms. Newington's part to get from "peanut" to "grapefruit," she managed to do it in a way that kept her father from becoming angered by his inability to find the word he wanted. At the same time, Ms. Newington knew that she had the advantage of living away from home and not having to talk with her father daily or hourly. "If I had to interpret what he said all the time," she commented, "I might lose my patience and say something like, 'Don't be silly! Nobody eats peanuts for breakfast,' instead of taking the time to find out what he was really trying to say."

The difficulties that occur when your relative has trouble in making himself understood are self-evident. He may forget names, mix reality with fantasy, ramble incoherently, make mistakes in word order, or repeat the same phrase over and over.

It is more problematic to determine if the impaired patient understands what is said to him. The same kinds of "scrambled connections" that interfere with his ability to communicate may also prevent him from understanding you. Although this can be extremely frustrating, and occasionally even dangerous to your patient, it has its humorous side:

MRS. LOUISE THOMAS: "You know, my husband can't do much of anything. He has two dental plates, an upper and a lower, and in the morning, before I give him his breakfast, he goes into the bathroom to get them. And he knows it's two, so he brings me two somethings, towels, or toothbrushes, or whatever, instead of the dental plates."

To give your relative a better chance of grasping what you are saying, and to improve your own chances of being understood, treat him like the unique individual he is. Address him by name and wait until you have his attention before you start to speak. Make sure your voice is loud enough to be audible. Allow time for your relative to understand your message. Repeat your communique if that seems necessary. Use brief and simple phrases and an easy vocabulary. Be tactful when it is necessary to correct his behavior.

Talk about things that interest your relative, about where you are going today, and what you are doing now. Don't talk to another person about your relative in his presence as if he weren't there.

You can reinforce your verbal message with nonverbal ones by pointing, gesturing, and using "body language" to convey your pleasure or displeasure with your relative's behavior. Soothing gestures, like calming words, mitigate tension and anger. They communicate love and understanding.

> MR. HORACE BEST: "Is it better to try to help? When my mother is trying to find a word for something, and she pauses, should I help her? Sometimes I say, 'I don't know what you're saying, try again,' or I give her a list of things, which might include the one she's referring to. I can't tell if it's better to help her, or if I should force her to exercise her memory. I don't know whether it is more frustrating to her to be told what she's thinking, or to me to wait while she searches her mind for the right word."

Mr. Best can solve his dilemma by supplying the word for his mother when she falters. He can also try to understand what she is saying by asking, "Do you mean . . . ?" or other leading questions similar to those used by Ms. Newington. His response in a given situation will depend on whether his mother seems agitated or relieved when he helps her complete a thought.

REPETITION

The patient who performs the same action over and over again becomes a great trial to the caregiver. The behavior is annoying to watch and, in public, it can cause embarrassment to the caregiver.

> MS. DOROTHY WEISS: "My father takes his shoes off, ties the shoelaces, and knots them. Then he ties the shoes together by the laces. And of course then he can't put the shoes back on. He will sit and do that for an hour."

Verbal repetition is irritating, too. One resourceful husband, whose wife kept asking the same questions over and over again ("What are we having for supper?" "Didn't we just have that yesterday?"), bought his wife a notebook. In it he wrote a simple meal plan and helped her to check off, every day each different menu.

> Ms. Beverly Ulrich: "I used to get very aggravated at my mother and say, 'You're so stubborn!' Then I'd realize that although I told her six times, each time she heard it, it was the first time. She's forgotten the other times. To me it's repetition, to her it's new information."

When the repetitious behaviors of your memory-impaired relative threaten to overwhelm your fortitude and patience, remember to take a few moments for yourself. Go into another room for a couple of minutes, pound a pillow, take a brisk walk around the block, or try one of the relaxation techniques we discuss in Chapter 6. Your ability to deal with your own frustrations and with your relative's behavior will be enhanced by refreshing yourself. Once you are revitalized and calmer, you may be able to devise your own solutions to these problems.

Fading In and Out of Lucidity

If your relative has a problem with attention, he may lose the thread of the conversation and stop talking in the middle of a sentence.

> Mr. Maxwell Whittaker: "My wife is sometimes lucid enough to be aware. She says she's trying to talk to me and nothing comes out right, and there's something terribly wrong, and won't I please help?
>
> "There are times when she's lucid and other times when she's not. She knows what's going on, but she can't concentrate. She doesn't have the ability to read, or watch television. I feel she should have some stimulation. That's why I read to her.
>
> "Sometimes when I say something to her, she won't understand what I'm saying, so I'll repeat it. Then she'll shake her head—she hasn't

173

absorbed it. However, the next day, or two days later, she'll refer to something that I had said to her when I felt I hadn't reached her at all."

When your family member has lapses of memory, your frustration may be so acute that your natural desire is to scold him. Instead, count to ten and try to refrain from criticizing him, which will only make things worse. Reacquaint your relative with the facts, and try to retrace steps with him.

Mr. Ira Fallon handled his dilemma with a sense of humor that always comes through for him in crisis situations. Mr. Fallon said to his impaired mother-in-law: "Let's see, where could you have put that curtain rod? The last time we saw it was when Ginger was here and took down the bathroom curtains to wash them." (The search begins.) He reports: "It's not in the bathroom, or the linen closet. It's not on the window or in the broom closet. Well" (to his mother-in-law), "don't worry" (mumbling "Damn, damn," under his breath), "we'll find it."

Later that evening, when Mr. Fallon went to the freezer to get some ice cream: "Well, of all things, look what's here!" (with amazement)— "the curtain rod!" His good-natured laughter has the ring of "Oh, my God, what will she do next?" When you can laugh about a memory lapse, perhaps that's the best remedy you can provide for yourself.

IF YOUR PATIENT BECOMES SILENT

We have discussed some of the problems in communication that can occur when your relative has lost a word or expression he wants to use or doesn't understand the meaning of what you tell him. Such difficulties may become more pronounced to the point where some victims of Alzheimer's disease and other similar illnesses simply stop talking.

MR. NORMAN LAWRENCE: "My sister doesn't speak very much. I try to talk to her. When you're all by yourself, you want to hear somebody's voice, but she won't say a word. She was always a quiet person, but now she hardly speaks at all. And at times, she seems to want to say something, but it's as if she's asleep while she's awake."

Such silence puts an additional burden on the caregiver. He must not only understand the patient's needs and respond to them without any clear communication from the patient, but also cope with the increased sense of isolation that results from that loss of communication. Try to remember that there is a great fund of nonverbal communication on which you can draw. Look for physical signs—smiles, nods of the head, touches of the hand, and eye movements are ways in which your patient may still signal his needs and his companionship.

Touching, hand-holding, and other forms of loving, nonverbal communication can help to reach someone whose power over words is diminished or whose way or receiving and processing information sometimes seems mysterious. It is always worth it to keep trying.

Use as many nonverbal clues as possible. An intuitive person can read someone's eyes or facial expression. Negative gestures such as a frowning face, tight jaw, or pursed lips are easy to interpret. Pacing, yelling, and banging communicate frustration and rage.

When your loved one shows distress or unhappiness by using such gestures, try to respond with as much delicacy as you are capable of. Soothe him and show that you are understanding and caring.

Sexual Communication

Patients with Alzheimer's disease or similar illnesses often desire and are capable of continued sexual communication and activity. Depending on the patient's relationship with a spouse and the feelings of the wife or husband, these needs may be met without incident. But sometimes the behaviors of the memory-impaired person are inappropriate. They may range from public disrobing (forgetting to dress and running out of the house without clothes) to indiscreet masturbation (usually fondling the genitals, which feels good to the patient).

175

Ms. MARGO GILLIAM: "I have a friend whose father has Alzheimer's disease. He's been living with her and her family for a few months, and when she calls me long-distance, I tell her jokingly that the telephone company is going to cut us off, because the conversation sounds obscene. She says that her father is constantly masturbating—anytime, all the time, anywhere in the house. It makes her very angry."

Many people report that their spouses show increased sexual desire, which may occur as a result of brain injury. They are sometimes annoyed by the demands of the Alzheimer's patient.

Ms. ANNE HOBART: "I work full-time, and every morning before I go to work I have to dress my husband and give him his breakfast. And every single morning while I'm helping him dress, he's trying to get me to have sex with him—stroking me, waving his penis at me. It's such a turnoff. All I want to do is get out of the house and get to work on time."

It is important to remember that a demand for sex may also be a desire for physical comfort and reassurance in the form of some bodily contact. Holding the person may be sufficient to satisfy the patient's need to be touched and the need for affection between the patient and the caregiver. In certain circumstances, this can be difficult to keep in mind:

MR. MARK PERRIN: "My brothers and sisters decided that Dad should have a vacation. He's been taking care of mother for nearly seven years without a break. So the five of us chipped in for a five-day trip to Mexico. Each of us paid a fifth of the fare and each of us took one day with Mom.

"I've never had such a shocking, humiliating experience in my life. My own mother tried to seduce me! Almost as soon as I arrived, she invited me to go to bed with her. We were planning to have a family dinner with my sister, but when Sis arrived, Mom said, 'We don't need other people—just the two of us—let's go into the bedroom and close the door. Come on, we don't need anyone else.'

"I blushed with shame. How could she say such things to me? On the other hand, I realized that I was nothing more than a substitute for Dad,

176

and since Dad's not around, she probably thinks that I'll do everything for her that Dad does. It made me so incredibly angry. Who does she think I am? I'm her son, not her husband! But it made me sad, too. I'm sure she was just looking for some reassurance and not sex at all. So I just told her not to worry, that everything would be all right and Dad would be home soon, and that meanwhile it was time for dinner. But as I patted her hand, I was still gulping because I was so alarmed."

Mr. Perrin was confused and angry at his mother's suggestion, although he recognized that she probably mistook him for his father and simply wanted some attention and reassurance. His ability to calm and distract his mother, despite his own embarrassment, saved the situation from becoming fraught with unnecessary tension.

Problems with Perception and Reality

Some people with Alzheimer's disease or other forms of memory loss develop false notions of reality. These may seem obviously foolish or inaccurate ideas to you, but your patient believes them with absolute certainty. Sometimes these misperceptions develop as a result of simple physical problems. For example, the older person whose hearing is poor may not be able to distinguish between your voice and a radio news report. Suddenly, your patient announces in panic, "There's a fire across the street!" The fire is across the street from the radio station, of course, but your patient's ears have confused the source of information. (This is another reason why regular medical checkups are important.)

People with Alzheimer's disease can't remember who people are, where their possessions are, or what anyone tells them. A memory-impaired person may imagine that people who are deceased are still alive. He may call for his mother, long dead, and insist that he can actually see her and speak with her.

MR. EDDIE OLINSKY: "My wife Maggie is always saying to me 'Where's Mama?' I say, 'She's in the kitchen,' or, 'She's shopping, she'll be back soon.' Sometimes, Maggie will pace around the room repeating 'When is Mama coming?' and I answer, 'She'll be here,' as soothingly as I can.

"At first I didn't know what to answer. I tried to be realistic. When she said, 'Where's Mama?' I would ask, 'What Mama?' and she would answer, 'My Mama.' Then I would tell her 'Your Mama's not here, she's gone.' But then she would panic, and become very anguished, and cry, 'Oh, where is she?'

"I saw that the truth was hurting her, and I didn't want to do that, and I didn't want her to panic. So now I say, 'Mama's going to come.' And if you believe in the spiritual life, it's not exactly a fib. Why tell Maggie the reality that her mother is dead, if it will only hurt and upset her? I just try to reassure her."

A Sense of Time Vanishes

Jess Walker had been an assistant vice president of a bank. At his retirement, after fifty years' service, he was given a gold watch that signified he had served the company well. Jess was 70 and looked forward to retirement. He and Abigail, his wife of thirty-two years, planned to travel to see their children and other friends and relatives. They did so until one day, in Arizona, Jess looked at his gold watch and couldn't figure out what the numbers meant. Having been a very orderly and punctual man all his life, Jess told Abigail that he was worried about being late for work. Abigail, alarmed, reminded her husband that he was no longer working and didn't have to worry about getting up or being at work on time. But Jess started getting up at all hours of the night and dressing to go to the office.

Later, when they returned home, Abigail took Jess to a neurologist because of his confused behavior and loss of memory. The neurologist told her that Jess's lost sense of time was the result of a loss in brain function and was seen often in patients with Alzheimer's disease. Jess's internal clock, which schedules eating, sleeping, and waking behaviors, was now disturbed, which is why he turned night into day.

All of us are dependent on external as well as internal clocks to routinize our lives and save us from excess preoccupation with getting places on time or overstaying our visits. The impaired person who, like Mr. Walker, has lost that sense of time will want to leave a place as soon as he gets there and will feel that he's been abandoned for hours when you've only been away a few minutes. In order to measure the passage of time, we need memory. When memory fades, the judgment that allows us to measure time spent or time passed also fades.

Abigail tried several things to put her husband's mind at rest. At home, she hid the clocks and his watch. When she visited her children, she would send her husband to the recreation room with his grandchildren. Jess loved to play cards. He would play cards with the boys while she visited with her daughter. It was a good arrangement; otherwise Jess would get restless and want to go home right away.

MR. SIMON BODINE: "When my uncle came to live with us, the first time I took him out driving, every time we saw a clock he would reset his watch, and then wind it. As we drove along, he would reset his watch, and then wind it. Finally, I said, 'Uncle Horace, let me fix it.' I set the watch correctly and gave it to him.

"Later that day, we went out again, and there he was with the watch, doing it all over again. I got so aggravated I was about to snatch it from him, when I took a good look and realized it wasn't the same watch! It turned out he had three of them, and to this day, whichever one he's wearing, he can't set it right.

"I hate the whole charade, but now, at least, I know what's going to happen. After all, it's just a little thing. In a way, my uncle's happiness is in those watches. If that's the most annoying thing he ever does, let him have them."

By indulging his uncle in this repetitive habit, Mr. Bodine is following our model of consistent, empathic responsiveness. As he says, he hates the constant repetitiveness, and he is frustrated by the fact that his uncle can never get the time set right. Yet, his loving attention makes his uncle's life, and his own, easier.

Clinging Behavior

MS. ROSALIE GEHRENS: "My husband is so possessive, I swear he's like my shadow. Where I go, he goes. If I'm out of the room, he comes searching for me in the other room. At night, when I bathe him and put him to bed nice and clean, he's so grateful and sweet. Then, I tell him, 'Now, you stay in bed quietly. I have to take my bath and get myself ready for bed.' He cannot even stay in bed that long. He's out, and in the bathroom, looking for me."

Clinging behavior on the part of the memory-impaired person can be very irritating and annoying to the caregiver who may not be able to bathe, sleep, relax, or even go to the bathroom without constantly being followed. What makes the confused person want to stick to you like glue? It no doubt stems from the insecurity that confronts him due to the loss of memory. To the memory-impaired person, like the infant in the crib who drops his toy and cries, out of sight is out of mind.

Patients who have an illness such as Alzheimer's disease are really cut off, because they can't trust to memory. In our healthy memories we can hold an image of someone that helps us to visualize what the person looks like and gives us a feeling of constancy even when he is absent. As a consequence of memory loss, your patient probably cannot retain a visual image of you. In your absence, he may even feel permanently abandoned. Your departure thus triggers feelings of insecurity.

There are several ways that caregivers have elected to deal with this problem. Mrs. Elise Monroe doesn't let it bother her. Her husband gets upset if she's gone for as little as ten or fifteen minutes. As often as she can, she takes him with her wherever she goes. He insists on coming with her, because he is worried about her getting lost. As she says, "I guess we worry about each other."

Mr. Arbolino diverts his sister so he has fifteen minutes to shower: "My sister wants to help me, but there isn't very much she can do. I let her grate bread crumbs from the stale Italian bread. I only give her three or four pieces, just enough for one meal. It's a small job. I give her the bread just before I take my shower because I know it will take her at least ten or fifteen minutes and she'll stay at it for that length of time. That's when I can disappear without her following me."

When you must leave your patient, try to reassure him that you will be back, say, at 5:00 PM. Draw a picture of a clock showing the time you'll return and leave that, with a big note saying, "I'll be back at 5," in a conspicuous place. If you can, call your relative while you are out and remind him that you'll be home soon. It may not work all of the time, but it will work some of the time, and making the effort will make you feel better. The key is to use whatever suggestions work for you.

Patients exhibit tremendous anxieties about being left alone by the caregiver, even for brief periods of time. This is true even when the caregiver is a home attendant whom the patient does not actually know well. That person—the one who feeds, dresses, supervises bathroom habits, and comforts the patient—comes to be viewed by the patient as his primary source of security. This may cause the patient's spouse or child to feel jealous, rejected, and resentful about the patient's seeming ingratitude for past dedication.

If you feel upset or become angry at what appears to be your relative's manifest disloyalty, remember that he is a victim of his own loss—that of memory—and as such is not consciously devaluing you or your services. He can't help himself, but you can: through trying to understand his behavior and your own reactions, you can soothe yourself and per-haps experience a minimum of discomfort in this situation.

Quality, Not Quantity, Counts!

It is really the quality of the relationship between you and your im-paired relative, rather than the amount of time that you spend together, that is significant. For example, you can spend the whole day in the house with your husband or wife and never say a word or even walk over to touch him or her; or you can be together for just a few hours, perhaps simply holding hands. Your own experience can demonstrate the difference in the degree of communication between these two exam-ples. When the major caregiver (whether child, or spouse, or sibling) is able to change his attitude toward the Alzheimer's victim, to become more positive, we can anticipate some changes in the behavior of the patient as well.

The quality of the time you spend with your impaired relative can be enhanced even though the changes in his behavior may be very small ones. The major change will be in your attitude toward the patient. And when you believe that such change is possible, the belief itself counteracts feelings of hopelessness and helplessness that are paralyzing.

One way to counteract those feelings is to use the "act like" approach. As we commented earlier, "acting like" we are attractive, self-confident, and successful will help to make us feel that way. Don't give in to laziness or apathy and stay in your pajamas all day. Resist the temptation to wear the same old housedress because you're not going out today. Your own good feelings about yourself will radiate to your patient and to others around you.

To help ensure that quality time, it's worth the effort to plan the hours you will spend with your relative. If he has enjoyed traveling, you may wish to organize one-day sightseeing or overnight trips for the two of you. The interest and enthusiasm that you show in the project will help spark his positive feelings.

Ms. Sophia Graziana: "Last year, my sister and I had a very good year. I was determined to make it good, and I worked hard. We went to Italy; we went to the Poconos; and we went to the White Mountains for weekends. She enjoyed the trips immensely. She remembered all our cousins, which was great. She was good! I said to myself, 'I'm not waiting until . . . .' This year, she's already deteriorated quite a bit. I'm glad I made the effort when I did."

RESTLESSNESS, AGITATION, AND RAGES

Ms. Carmelita Dworkin: "My mother builds up a tremendous amount of agitation and races from one end of the house to the other, looks out of the window, as if to satisfy herself, then comes back. And no matter what the weather—heat, cold, even heavy rain—she goes out and walks. Walking with her is real exercise. She'll walk your legs off!"

Restlessness, another characteristic behavior of the victims of Alzheimer's disease, is probably due to organic changes. Children who have some organic impairment, even of a minimal nature, exhibit similar characteristics. They become hyperactive and disorganized. The same kind of behavior is seen in older people who suffer from memory impairment.

> Ms. Maria Quinones: "My cousin has never said anything to me about her condition, but she told her brother that she knows there is something wrong with her. I believe that, because from time to time she will begin to cry, for no apparent reason, with deep, heavy sobs that go on and on. I wonder if this violent crying is a sign that she's angry with herself, or that she knows that there's something wrong and she can't do anything about it."

The patient's concern about his disability may account for his irritation. At some (perhaps preconscious) level, he is aware of being different from before. He may recognize that he is not behaving like most people but doesn't know why or how to change. When patients verbalize their awareness that they are not the same as they once were, it is painful both to the patient and to the caregiver.

Victims of Alzheimer's disease and similar illnesses may suddenly erupt into violent and irrational rages. These rages do not seem related to external events, nor to another person's provocation. Caregivers have described experiences in which confused relatives spat at them, pinched or punched them, or threatened to hit them with books, lamps, or kitchen implements.

A patient may angrily fire a homemaker or health aide who has been helping in the house for many months. He may furiously accuse a spouse of betrayal, or of being an imposter.

Was the memory-impaired person distressed about not being able to remember his life? Angry at the attendant? Trying to get even with the caregiver for leaving him alone? It may be all or none of these reasons that provoke a patient's rage. One of the common symptoms of Alzheimer's and other similar diseases is emotional instability, in which heightened, intensified, easily-upset feelings are the rule.

These rages are not well understood since the patient cannot tell us what he is feeling or what precipitated his aggressive actions. It is unfortunate that we do not know the precise source of the patient's anger. However, psychologists speculate that such rages are due to unconscious fears, and the patient's reaction to his own inabilities to communicate or to do things for himself. These catastrophic reactions may also be caused by brain damage.

What is extremely important is that you, the caregiver, not be the physical object of the patient's rage. Should there be an imminent danger or threat of physical harm to you, you must leave the scene of danger at once, so as not to be injured.

Go to a neighbor and call the local hospital. (Some hospitals, such as Beth Israel in New York City, have an "Alzheimer's unit." They will send an ambulance with attendants who are prepared to handle the enraged patient. If your city does not have such a service, suggest one to the local hospital administrator.) If it is avoidable, try not to involve the police, whose presence can be embarrassing to you. Although some police units have special training and are helpful, in general police personnel may not be as well equipped as hospital paramedics are to handle the patient.

When your patient is once again calm, and it is safe for you to return, don't mention the incident. This may be difficult, because family members may take the patient's rage personally, even though it may have nothing to do with them, Most likely, the patient won't remember the incident anyway. Here, loss of memory works in your favor. Try to forget the incident, but stay alert to the fact that it could happen again, and that you must first protect yourself and get out of the line of fire. Then make sure that the patient is protected from himself.

While it may be impossible to determine what triggers an angry tantrum in your memory-impaired relative, we have learned something about the way certain situations tend to affect people with this handicap.

For example, Ralph Crown's father was only mildly impaired when the Crowns had a week-long family reunion. Ralph's brother George and his family came from across town, and his sister Teri, who was her father's favorite, brought her husband and children all the way from Texas. The second evening, as they were all sitting down to dinner, the elder Mr. Crown returned from his daily walk, looked around, and hollered, "What is everybody doing here? You were just here the other day! Why don't you go home?" Ralph was shocked that his father would say something like that, especially to Teri, after she had travelled hundreds of miles to see him.

Ms. Angie Calmirras knows she can't leave her brother alone. When she goes out, she always asks one of her friends to come and stay with him. Recently, her friend Lila came to dinner, and planned to stay with her brother while Angie went to her Great Books group.

After dinner, another friend came to pick Angie up for the meeting. Suddenly, her brother made a nasty scene, shouting, "You're trying to take my money away from me! You're trying to take my business away from me! You're trying to throw me out of my own company! All of you, right now, get out!"

Angie felt very bad, even though she knew friends understood because she had told them all about her brother's illness. Still, she was afraid to let Lila remain in the house, so she stayed home from the meeting.

In both these situations, the rage may have been triggered by too many people and too much noise. That could have contributed to the confusion and irritability that led to heightened aggression.

Even the most minute change may lead to additional confusion and disorientation in the patient. When strangers are around, the patient may also feel ignored and become very aggressive. Paying consistent attention to him usually elicits positive responses from him.

Although many of the furious outbursts that we see in memory-impaired patients have no apparent cause, some, unfortunately, seem to be provoked either by a frustrated caregiver or in response to some unresolved difficulty in the past, before the patient became ill. A woman who was in the care of a son-in-law whom she had never liked slammed a door in his face. A husband spat at the wife who belittled him when he failed to remember a word he wanted. When her husband tried to hurry her out of bed one morning, a confused wife kicked him so hard that she raised welts on his arm.

Earlier, we talked about the many ways in which this illness generates angry feelings in the caregivers who must watch as their loved ones change and deteriorate. We stressed your need to manage your own very understandable angry reactions, partly because anger tends to beget anger. Your outburst can trigger one in your patient, as can your teasing, or impatience, or resentment. The more you can understand, accept, and manage your own angry feelings, the less chance you will have of provoking angry feelings in your loved one, and the more creativity you will be able to apply to discovering and relieving the sources of his anger.

> MR. GEORGE KELLERMAN: "Every morning, my wife would start off the day by fighting with me. I couldn't understand it. I finally figured out that she was having bad dreams during the night and I was appearing in those dreams. She would wake up in the morning and we would start fighting, and I wouldn't know where it was coming from.
>
> "I gave her a piece of lined paper on a clipboard, and on top of the page I wrote, 'I am angry with George because . . . ,' and I told her to fill in the lines. Now, at least, she doesn't begin the day by picking a fight."

Our model for living with an impaired relative is one of consistent, empathic responsiveness. Think about how you like to be treated, and what it must be like to be in the position of the patient. As a model, it is an ideal to strive toward. Being human, we cannot hope to be tuned in every minute of the day to the needs of the impaired person. However, we can try to adopt an attitude of empathy, so that even at times when we run out of patience and give vent to our own frustration, irritability, or anger, we can come back to a better understanding of ourselves as well as of others.

HALLUCINATIONS

Hallucinations are perceptions of external objects that are not present in the environment. Although most hallucinations are "seen" or "heard," any of the senses may be involved.

MR. CURTIS JENNER: "My uncle complains constantly that his clothing is damp. He takes off his underwear and lays it on the radiator, saying, 'Damp, damp, damp!' Everything is damp. It feels moist to him, although it really isn't. He will mop his face and head with tissue after tissue, even though he seems to the rest of us to be thoroughly dry. We don't understand why he has this feeling of being perpetually damp. My aunt speculates that it's because he is taking medication for his heart condition, but the cardiologist never told us that this medicine would make him feel sweaty when he isn't."

Actually, hallucinations are sensations that arise within the patient himself. A hallucination may terrify the patient if he smells fire, or shadowboxes with his own image on the wall because he thinks it's someone else. If he has a conversation with a stranger in the mirror (himself) or thinks he sees a welcome friend, he may be amused by the hallucination.

MS. VIRGINIA ELGIN: "Right now my mother is in a stage in which she talks to herself. She goes to the mirror and if I ask her, 'What are you doing?' she'll say, 'I'm talking to myself.' Sometimes, instead of the mirror, she'll go to the bookcase and talk to that.

"From time to time, while she's talking, I hear a very sensible conversation, not the confused gibberish she talks most of the time. She says, 'My hair is terrible today.' (She was always vain.) 'So I think I'll wait for my daughter to come home. She'll take me to the beauty parlor.'"

Ms. Elgin must sometimes feel drained and saddened by her mother's confusion and lost abilities. She has, however, reacted to her mother's need to look as attractive as possible by having her hair done and trying to help her with her grooming. Responding, when possible, to the feelings that may have inspired a hallucination is probably the best way to handle it.

DELUSIONS

Your confused patient may express thoughts that are actually delusions. A delusion is a belief that can be shown to be contrary to fact. For example, your relative may complain that people who are persecuting him are in the next apartment, though the apartment next door is empty. He may declare that the people in the television set are talking about him in derogatory terms, although the set is off and the room is quiet.

SUSPICIOUSNESS

Forgetful people have a tendency to be somewhat paranoid or suspicious of others. Because they can't find their money, keys, glasses, bankbooks, and other possessions (having either forgotten where they've put them or hidden them so well no one can find them), they may assume that these things have been stolen. Calls to the police accusing close friends and relatives of stealing are quite frequent. The affections of dearest relatives are often alienated when these events occur.

Ms. JILL SWENSON: "My father doesn't make sense out of anything. He's got this hang-up with money. He's especially disturbed about the few dollars that he inherited from his father. His father died about twenty years ago, but somehow it got locked up in Father's mind that he's afraid we're spending the money. We keep trying to tell him, 'Don't worry, Dad, the money is safe in the bank.' "

Trying to reason with Mr. Swenson further compounds his daughter's distress. It is fruitless to argue. In a similar situation, try to deflect the issue by showing him the bankbook and saying, in a reassuring tone, "We will help you to protect your money." If that doesn't work, try to distract the patient by asking him to do a simple chore, look at a photo album, or go for a walk. The topic may come up again, so be prepared not to take the accusations personally. They are the result of feelings of loss and confusion emanating from the damage to the brain.

Ultimately, taking away valuables like jewelry and keeping spare sets of keys and eyeglasses will help to avoid awkward confrontations.

We grow up with a healthy sense of cynicism and disbelief. We learn to check out our suspicions for they are sometimes based on fact. While a memory-impaired person may seem overly suspicious, don't automatically dismiss his concern—it may be founded on fact.

Mr. William Harrison, who suffers from Alzheimer's disease, claimed that he had spent several sleepless nights in a row. His wife Nora had left him in their apartment with a home attendant (a woman who had been hired on the strength of recommendations but without written references) while she worked nights in a hospital emergency room. Nora Harrison could not understand her husband's claim of alertness, since he was supposed to receive a sleeping pill before bedtime. One evening Mrs. Harrison came home early and found the attendant asleep while her husband was awake and agitated. Her unexpected arrival revealed that the attendant was taking the sleeping pills and getting a good night's sleep, while her husband remained agitated and sleepless. Needless to say, Mr. Harrison's "suspicions" were well founded and the attendant was discharged.

Excess suspiciousness causes people to overreact to situations that may be benign.

Ms. Ada Wesley had been walking on a school street at noon when the youngsters were coming out of school for lunchtime. The noise and hordes of children confused her. Fearful of being followed by some teenage girls, Ms. Wesley clutched her purse to her breast. Her suspicion changed to panic when the girls suddenly seemed to be directly behind her. She started to scream and, in her confusion, ran right into them. The girls were alarmed and yelled at her, "You're a crazy lady!" Her fears of being a victim of a mugging caused her to become more disoriented and confused and compounded her suspiciousness, which then brought about overreaction. The girls felt unjustly accused; thus, their cries of "crazy lady."

When excess suspicion causes our confused loved one to blame us erroneously for imagined evils, our anger wells up, and we feel abused by his false accusations. It is difficult to remember that the accusation stems from fear and from the inability to test reality. For the person who cannot remember what happened an hour ago, or even who he is, there is no place to feel safe. Overwhelming feelings of loss and distress cause him to feel terribly small, diminished, and vulnerable. Caregivers often react to the suspicions of a confused person by feeling hurt. Because the impaired person looks and sometimes sounds reasonable, it is hard for us to believe that the suspicious behavior is beyond control. In fact, the patient is struggling to make sense of nonsense in a world that is unfamiliar, terribly disorienting, and frightening. He needs all the reassurance you can give him.

Depression and Memory Impairment

MRS. FORREST: "I know that my husband has memory impairment. He won't remember when he gets up in the morning what day of the week it is—'Is it Sunday?' 'Is it Tuesday?'—but later on in the day he'll seem to be more aware of what day it is and where things are. And he's often very agitated in the mornings. During the day he calms down. He even takes a little nap in the afternoon. But as night comes on, he'll begin pacing again, back and forth, back and forth.

"I thought those behaviors were just part of the condition. But my doctor asked me to watch him, to see if I saw any change in his behavior during the course of the day.

"The doctor told me that his agitated behavior could be a sign of depression. That surprised me. I kept saying that he wasn't depressed, because I figured that 'depressed' meant being very unhappy, not moving, not being interested in anything. But my doctor said there is such a thing as an agitated depression, when the patient shows a great deal of activity and nervous energy. He said that people who are depressed experience it most keenly in the morning. So it seems my husband is depressed as well as memory-impaired."

Mr. Forrest's dual affliction is not that unusual. Patients who have suffered some memory loss may become depressed as a result of being aware of their forgetfulness. They may be responding to their consequent feelings of loss of ability and self-esteem. They may also become depressed as a result of another unrelated loss: the death of a close friend, spouse, or other relative, for example.

Moreover, recent research indicates that over 10 percent of the patients who have been diagnosed as having organically based senile dementia are actually suffering primarily from depression, and in some cases, from depression alone, with no organic involvement.

How can you tell the difference between depression and an organic cause of forgetfulness in your patient? The two diseases are often confused, yet it is important to distinguish one from the other, both for your relative's sake and for your own. How much of the Alzheimer's patient's illness is due to organic damage, and how much to depression? Can the depression be treated? How can you, the caregiver, keep from becoming depressed as you cope with your loved one's problems?

MR. WARREN: "Two years ago, my mother was having blackouts—not lengthy ones, but enough to concern us. So Dad and I took her to a neurologist who did some tests and said that she had some arterial blockage, so that it was reasonable to expect to see some memory impairment in her.

"But since my father died, a year ago, she has become so much worse that I took her back to the neurologist. She had already seen a psychologist. Mother was very well behaved for the psychologist, very rational, and seemed not to show the kind of distress I see in her all the time—she cries, is apathetic, sits for hours, and she needs somebody to tell her when and how to do every little thing.

"The neurologist kept saying, 'Oh, yes, there's definite organic damage, no question about it.' I asked him what he thought caused it. He said,

'You can call it senile dementia, or Alzheimer's disease, or whatever the fashion is today, but as far as I'm concerned, it's just accelerated aging. But there's been no radical change—she has exactly the same amount of damage as she had two years ago.'

"But Doctor,' I said, 'She acts like a completely different person!'

"He didn't really have much to say about that.

"So I took her back to the psychologist again. This time, at least, the psychologist was able to draw her out, and she said some things that worry me: 'I want to be dead!' 'I'm losing my mind. I'm afraid I'll be sent to a mental hospital.' She was wringing her hands and crying.

"Is she depressed? Is it arteriosclerosis? Is she still mourning my father? Is she upset because she's aware of the changes in her behavior as a result of the stroke? I don't know, but her crying and her telling me she wants to die make me feel depressed, too!"

Patients who have had strokes suffer from depression that appears to be related to the level and severity of the impairment sustained by the stroke. The depression may appear from six months to two years after the stroke has happened.

For example, impairment that is associated with different lesions may be implicated in mood disorders. It has been found that catastrophic and depressive reactions occur more frequently among patients whose left brain is damaged (about 79 percent) as opposed to those people whose right brain is affected. The left hemisphere of the brain is generally thought to control reading, writing, and arithmetic skills and memory, while the right side of the brain involves spatial and artistic intelligence. Those who suffer severe aphasia (loss of the facility for understanding written or verbal language) appear depressed after they have repeatedly failed in their attempts to communicate. Thus mood disorder seems to be a specific complication of stroke, not merely a response to a motor disability.

The use of antidepressant medications such as tricyclic antidepressants in the treatment of poststroke depression victims is effective in some cases, although each case must be considered individually. After about one month, personality is often restored, and the patient seems less irritable and shows interest in other people, as well as improved concentration and attention.

SYMPTOMS OF DEPRESSION

Is your relative sad or apathetic? Or does he become manic (hyperactive) and magnify physical complaints, or act hypochondriacal—that is, take unnecessary pills for imaginary ailments? Does he lack appetite, complain of indigestion and constipation?

Does he have problems sleeping? For example, does he awaken early in the morning, usually between 2:00 and 4:00 AM, complaining of discomfort, anxiety, and worry, and find himself unable to return to sleep? Symptoms of sleep disturbance are common signs of depression.

Does your relative seem to have suicidal tendencies? Does he overmedicate himself? Does he drink and drive? Or drink and take drugs? Has he expressed a wish to kill himself? If so, his depression may be so severe that he may need to be hospitalized.

Every depressed person should be treated by a competent and qualified professional psychologist, psychiatrist, psychotherapist, or psychoanalyst.

Although some depressed people exhibit a temporary loss of memory for events, the symptom of memory loss is sometimes less evident in depression than the other symptoms we have mentioned. However, the major factor in a diagnosis of Alzheimer's disease or similar organically based illnesses is the loss of recent memory (memory for recent events). This capacity seems to be among the first to deteriorate, along with the abilities to learn new information, manipulate numbers, and keep track of personal possessions.

Does your relative seem to have mood swings, changes in feelings and emotions, and poor judgment? Is he disoriented as to time, place, and person—that is, does he know what day it is, where he is, and who you are? Is he confused? If some or all of these signs are present, then the person is probably organically impaired.

It is important to distinguish between a diagnosis of depression and one of Alzheimer's or other similar diseases. Organic damage to the brain is irreversible and untreatable, while depression is both treatable and reversible, through psychotherapy, often in combination with anti-depressant drugs prescribed by physician.

DRUGS AND ALCOHOL

Mood-altering drugs or alcohol may seem to offer relief to the depressed person, but their effects are short-lived and eventually backfire. Although tranquilizers or amphetamines may help ease a depression temporarily, they can lead to dependency and further impairment. Alcohol, while it may act as a quick stimulant, is in fact a long-term central nervous system depressant; any relief from alcohol is temporary.

Thus both the medicine cabinet and the liquor closet may be sources of increased depression for an already depressed person. Consequently, behavior that mimics organic confusion can occur when one is depressed. As suggested previously, taking several different medications can complicate either depression or a memory-impairing disease and can produce symptoms of mental confusion.

Alcoholics who develop memory impairment are affected by smaller amounts of alcohol than those people who drink only occasionally. Because alcoholics are often undernourished, their ability to function adequately is considerably decreased, and they exhibit behavior that is nasty and obnoxious. Alcohol only further confuses the Alzheimer's patient.

The primary concern of the caregiver must be to stop the supply of alcohol. In order to accomplish this and to manage the behavior of the alcoholic who is suffering from confusion and memory loss, he may need the help of a professional counselor experienced in alcohol addiction.

APATHY, ANTAGONISM, SADNESS

Coldness, moodiness, and lack of feeling for others or excess concern for himself are often characteristics of the Alzheimer victim's behavior. It is extremely painful to you as the caregiver to be so ill used; such self-absorption doesn't endear your patient to you after you have expended so much energy on his care. Perhaps you will be comforted to know that this type of behavior is due to the patient's constant fear. The confusion and disorientation that result from the damage to his brain make him fearful and self-absorbed. Although you are affected by the coldness, it is not really directed at you or meant to be hurtful.

THREAT OF SUICIDE

MR. IRA MORGAN: "I often wonder how much of my sister's condition is due to depression. She doesn't say, 'I'm depressed,' but she seems to be hurt by her son. She used to live with him, but one of his children was in an auto accident, and he found that his wife couldn't take care of both the child and my sister. So my nephew sent my sister to me.

"Once in a while, when we've been out for a walk, she'll be fine until we get home, and then she will begin to cry uncontrollably. I worry that she might make herself sick. She cries and cries and calls for her son Tommy. He's a good son, and he calls her up nearly every day.

"At one point he had to take her bankbooks away from her, and the car keys, because she really couldn't manage anymore. I'm not even sure that she knows what he did, or that she misses driving the car or keeping her checkbook. But I'm also not sure that she doesn't. I don't know what she feels. I can only speculate that if I had been told I wasn't capable of driving or of paying my bills anymore, I'd be pretty upset about it.

"It bothers me very much that she cries all the time and asks for Tommy, while it doesn't seem to matter that I'm the one who is here and taking care of her. In the beginning I used to scream at her, but that didn't help. Now, when I see her crying and rocking back and forth, it just destroys me."

If your relative cries a lot, or gets agitated and wails hysterically, or wants to cry but can't, it is okay to encourage tears but not to excess. While crying can be relieving, it also taxes the patient's energy, allowing less stamina with which to combat depressed feelings. If the person cannot stop crying, you might tell him to go ahead and cry but to look you straight in the eyes at the same time. Take his hand gently and coax him to look at you. It is not possible to cry and look someone in the eyes at the same time. If you repeat this several times, he will generally stop crying.

There are other ways in which you can mitigate the effects of sadness and depression on your patient and improve his sense of well-being.

When your relative becomes anxious, don't remind him of things in the future, even if they are joyous occasions, for the contrast to his own present state of joylessness may be too much to bear. Deal only with the here and now.

If your relative says he's afraid to be alone, take his alarm seriously. It is helpful if a neighbor or good friend or relative is able to stay with the patient until he is more at ease. Sometimes, however, distracting your patient and offering reassurance by your physical presence may be the only way to help him until he is once again in control of himself. Neither morning goodbyes, words of endearment and devotion, nor frequent reassuring telephone calls may be sufficient until the crisis is over.

With relatives and friends, organize a routine in which to complete the day's activities. This can be extremely helpful in motivating the memory-impaired, depressed patient when he has "slowed down." Following an organized routine will help your patient to restore his sense of self-esteem.

Make decisions for your patient when his depression impedes his ability to do so. Give him properly matching clothes when he can't choose what to wear. If you plan an event, simply take your impaired relative with you instead of forcing him to consider whether he will go or not. Do not rely on the judgment of someone who is both memory-impaired and depressed. The family must take over.

If your patient becomes agitated because you are in charge, try to stay calm and to divert him. Create an atmosphere of tranquility through subdued lights, soft background music on the radio, a quiet room. Talk to your family member in a quiet, slow, and calm way to preserve an attitude of mental calmness.

Arrange low-key activities, such as a walk through the park, a brief visit to one friend, or a movie, but avoid crowds and anything that is hurried or has any tension attached to it.

A depressed person does not benefit from the "pull yourself up by your bootstraps" philosophy that well-meaning friends so often use to try to mobilize him. Yelling at your patient, or telling him to "cut out the nonsense and get back to normal," or "do it and do it now," or the attitude of "a kick in the pants," is unhelpful. Competing with him for attention by letting him know his depression is "too much" for you to bear is really a demand that he get well in a hurry. Usually such an approach intensifies the unhappy patient's guilt feelings and his depression.

The depressed person feels all alone with his suffering. He may be fearful that, acting on impulse, he will harm himself. Even though he doesn't really want to die, he may have a premonition about his own death. If you sense that this is happening to your patient, it is important to be truthful with him. If you think that he can understand, explain that depression is an illness in which the nervous system does not function properly. Thoughts of death may become an obsession when a person's spirits are low and he feels sad; he may become afraid. It is important to remind him that when he feels better he doesn't dwell on thoughts of death. When the depression is lifted, such obsessive thoughts will disappear. If your patient seems well, then relapses, as do most patients, go through the same explanation each time the fears are mentioned. Each time you do so, the fears will diminish.

A crucial sign of trouble is your relative's expression of suicidal ideas.

Ms. Marilyn Elledge: "I belong to a support group for families of patients with Alzheimer's disease. But my brother Frank, who is the one who's sick, gives me a real hard time when it's time for me to go to the meetings. We have a senior citizen's center nearby, and one of the men there has offered to keep Frank company. When I told Frank this morning that it was time to leave, he started blaming me for the way he feels and the way he is, telling me that it's all my fault. He said that I'm going to drive him to suicide. I felt so terrible. I just sat down and cried."

If your patient has spoken of suicide, tight security and the help of family members is essential; the person should not be left alone. A suicidal patient usually wants to be left alone to make a suicide attempt. The rising tension and loss of hope is what precipitates most suicide attempts. Until the depressed person is treated and well on his way to recovery from the depression, he should be considered self-destructive. It is important to remind the depressed person that depressions come in cycles, but they are also self-limiting, and that eventually he will feel better.

Therapy for the Alzheimer's Patient

Some patients with mild forms of memory impairment benefit from memory enhancement programs in which they learn skills to improve their memories. They may also benefit from individual psychotherapy in the early stages of the illness, especially if they are suffering from anxiety and depression. Depression can be lifted through psychotherapy as the patient learns how he may be interfering with his own ability to improve his functioning.

Mrs. Herzog, a 62-year-old university professor, was experiencing some memory difficulties. She had problems in spelling and couldn't concentrate on preparing her lectures. Mrs. Herzog became anxious each time she sat alone to write.

In talking about her anxieties, she also recounted her youthful experiences as a victim of the Nazi holocaust. She recalled having felt severe separation anxiety because her mother was sent for several months to Treblinka, a Nazi prison camp. Later she and her mother were again separated from a beloved aunt and a grandmother. Now, at 62, Mrs. Herzog was planning to retire, and once again separation loomed large in her life. She would be separated from the career she had enjoyed for thirty years, her students, and fellow professors.

Through psychotherapy, she was able to link the two separations together. Mrs. Herzog can now separate out past anxieties and deal better with her current fears. She also practices memory training in her psychotherapy sessions. Her shame about being too small to help her family as a child and her current shame about having memory problems brings her a great deal of anxiety. Helping Mrs. Herzog to realize she is not responsible for either event and need not feel ashamed of herself will relieve her anxiety. Along with memory enhancement she will be enabled to cope with her diagnosis of Alzheimer's disease and her subsequent retirement.

While guilt and anger turned against the self have been believed to be the root of much depression in patients, more recently an understanding of shame and its role in depression has become a focus of psychotherapy. Shame-sensitive patients need an emotionally responsive therapist whose attitude and personality will help to heal the toxic shame of emotional abandonment. Adults are ashamed usually because they have been abandoned by caretakers in the past. In the present, the patient needs a compassionate caregiver who can focus on what the patient does that is healthy and right. "Catch me doing something right," is a good phrase to remember, helping us to believe and trust in our own goodness and to be more hopeful about ourselves and our lives.

Unfortunately, very few psychotherapy programs are available for the mildly impaired patient, and fewer therapists have the training in gerontology, compassion, and hopeful attitudes that would enable them to meet the needs of these patients.

In some day care centers and nursing homes, "reality orientation" is practiced. The goal of such treatment is to help the patient function better and, if possible, to prevent further decline.

In reality orientation, the patient's attention is frequently directed to a reality board on which are displayed in large numbers and letters the day of the week, the date, and other relevant facts. Guided in the relearning process, some patients may reinforce the everyday skills they already possess, like setting a table, making a sandwich, playing a game, or writing a postcard. The training is both therapeutic and stimulating to the patient. Although controversial, reality orientation is regarded as one way of maintaining the patient's interest in his surroundings and encouraging continued independent functioning. Reality orientation also promotes social interaction between patients, which is very beneficial.

Too often, well-meaning relatives (or staff members in a nursing home) encourage the patient's dependence by doing everything for him. Nursing home staff members are usually well-intentioned and find it easier to "mother" the elderly patient as one would a small child. However, it is known that overprotection by the well-meaning mother can foster lifelong dependency in a child; for the older adult, it may hasten his deterioration and subsequent decline.

CHAPTER 12

Everyday Life with the Alzheimer's Patient

*T*he purpose of this chapter is to alert you, the caregiver, to some of the difficulties you may encounter in caring for your memory-impaired relative, and to offer our best advice and the advice of other caregivers in coping with the hardships that brain failure can impose. Our motto is: "Forewarned is forearmed." Not every impaired person will behave in the same way as the people you will read about here. Each person with Alzheimer's disease or another variety of memory loss is an individual whose symptoms, while similar, may manifest themselves differently and in varying degrees. Some people deteriorate gradually, others rapidly. No one person will have every problem discussed here.

Remember that because he is ill, his human needs for love, attention, caring, and kindness may be intensified. He may still have a sense of humor and be able to enjoy life. Remember, too, that you are human also, and that, along with your caring and devotion, you will be subject to feelings of anger, unfairness, depression, guilt, and resentment at the enormous burdens you face.

Your common sense, good humor, and imagination will help you to get through critical moments and to find innovative solutions to problems that seem insoluble. Even small creative changes may enhance your daily life and help you to make the necessary adaptations that will comfort and sustain you and your patient.

Predictability is an important key to day-to-day living with a memory-impaired person. A structured environment and routines that don't change offer your patient a necessary feeling of comfort and security, and safety from physical hazards. Although it is extremely difficult, you must accept the fact that some capacities and skills that your impaired relative once possessed are permanently lost. Simplified tasks and activities will help him focus on the skills he still has rather than on those he has lost, and will therefore help maintain his self-respect.

You can also try breaking down necessary tasks step by step into their most elementary components. Systematizing the task in this way makes it easier to follow. For example, brushing one's teeth requires:

1. Picking up the toothbrush
2. Putting toothpaste on the brush
3. Inserting the brush into the mouth and brushing
    a. on the upper left side
    b. on the upper right side
    c. on the lower left side
    d. on the lower right side
    e. across the front top
    f. across the front bottom
4. Lowering the brush from the mouth
5. Spitting
6. Rinsing the mouth with water
7. Rinsing the brush
8. Putting the brush away

A patient may not be capable of doing a task entirely by himself but could pick up the sequence of steps. For example, you could break down brushing the patient's hair into these steps:

1. Put the brush in the patient's hand
2. Lift the patient's hand and brush to his head
3. Hold the patient's hand and gently run the brush through his hair, stroking gently, pulling down and out
   a. right side
   b. center right
   c. center left
   d. left side
   e. front
   f. back

If the patient seems ready to try brushing his own hair, let him try. Compliment his ability and how well he looks.

Your relative may sustain certain personality changes that lead him to overreact to situations. His volatility may seem like stubbornness, arbitrariness, or just plain orneriness, but it is often due to rapidly changing moods. These moods may be brought on by the unfamiliarity of a new situation, by confusion aroused by too large a group of people, or by his inability to do an apparently simple task that he finds extremely difficult. Swearing, sobbing, and physical or verbal aggression are typical overreactions to basic requests to eat, go to sleep, take a bath, or take a medication. Sometimes these reactions seem to have no apparent cause.

Consider that our familiar world has become strange and perhaps threatening to the person with brain damage, who can not manage to react in an ordinary way to an ordinary situation. Simplify, simplify, simplify, as you would for a brain-injured child. Consistent behavior is important. Do your best to contain your fears and your desire to shout or pout. If your relative overreacts or has an angry outburst, don't try to argue or to reason logically. Maintain a quiet, deliberate facade (despite your inner fears or rage), take several deep breaths, and try to pacify and mollify your upset relative. Take his hand gently and speak softly. When his overreaction has subsided, do whatever you need to do (talk to a friend, meditate, get some exercise) to relieve your own frustration and sadness. Use the tension-relieving exercises offered in Chapter 6.

Household Bywords: Safety and Structure

The home of a memory-impaired elderly person must be accident-proofed for his safety. Memory-impaired people are unable to protect themselves from household hazards because they have forgotten how. Consider the hazards in your own home:

- Are electric appliances such as irons, hair dryers, sewing machines, and electric saws and drills under lock and key?
- Do you keep medicines, household cleaners, and other dangerous substances in cabinets out of sight and out of reach?
- Have you concealed any exposed pipes, the hot water heater, and access to the furnace?
- Are extension cords and slippery rugs tacked down or removed?
- Are fragile knick-knacks and valuable antiques put away?

In addition, the older person needs bright lighting, conveniently placed handrails, and stairs with both reflector treads and a gate at the top. An older person may not only have problems with disorientation and balance; he may also be struggling with poor eyesight, reduced hearing, arthritis, vertigo, or any one of several other conditions that restrict safe, free movement.

For the older caregiver, problems with walking, balance, and falling can present further difficulties. The elderly spouse or sibling needs as much bodily protection as the patient.

MRS. STEEGER: "My husband is now in the stage of his illness where he has developed a fear of falling, just like an infant. It's a terrible feeling, the fear of falling. Even if you put him near a chair, and you point out to him, 'Look, the chair is here, just sit yourself down,' well, he grabs. He grabs onto me, even though I try not to hold him. He's so afraid of falling backwards into the chair that it takes fifteen minutes to sit him down.

"In the bathroom, he breaks everything he grabs onto to hold himself from falling. He grabbed onto the shower curtain and pulled the rod right down. I have more repair bills!"

The bathroom and the kitchen are perhaps the most dangerous rooms in the house. Mrs. Steeger might reduce her husband's tendency to pull on the shower curtain if she installed support bars for him to hold, such as those provided for the handicapped in public places.

Other bathroom safety aids include bright lights, a skid-proof mat in the bathtub, and good overflow drains in the tub and the sink, so that if the forgetful person leaves the water running, no flood will result.

In the kitchen, sharp knives and other dangerous kitchen implements should be out of sight and out of reach—an impaired person may forget how to use such tools safely. Take the knobs off the stove and put away the matches to avoid a serious fire hazard. Or, if you have a gas range, Mr. Kreuzer's solution might help you:

"My wife kept going into the kitchen, putting on a saucepan of water to heat for tea, turning on the burner, and forgetting all about it. Sometimes she would turn the gas burner on first and then forget to put the pot of water on it. She would do that at night, too—a cup of tea was her cure for insomnia.

"It certainly didn't cure mine! Every time she woke up, I woke up, too, to make sure she didn't burn the house down. After arguing and pleading with her not to turn on the gas in the middle of the night, one day I had an inspiration. I bought an asbestos mat that covered the top of the stove. It worked like a charm. She went near it once, and said, 'What's this?' I said, 'Just so you won't be making tea in the middle of the night.' She hasn't done it since."

Locks on exterior doors should be placed either at the top or the bottom, out of reach of the impaired person. Outside your house, entrances, stairways, and sidewalks should be brightly lit. If you have a swimming pool, it should be securely fenced with a locked gate, for even good swimmers can lose their memory of the skill:

> MR. MORRISON: "Last year my father would swim, but not for long. Now he can't even remember how to swim. I had to keep coaxing him into the water. I said, 'Sure, come on, like me. Just swim to me, from there to here.' He did it, but he didn't stay in the water long. I was just as glad—I had to stop and think to be sure that I could protect him in the water."

In addition to physical hazards, there is an invisible danger in some households. A direct correlation exists between rising tensions and a heightened number of accidents in the home. Therefore, make your home accident-proof first by decreasing any tension that may exist. Avoid a serious accident either by changing your pace (do things more slowly) or by modifying the atmosphere in your environment. Take time to release your own tensions, lest they contribute to emotional chilliness or outright hostility between you and your impaired relative.

IF YOUR RELATIVE FALLS DOWN

During the later phases of his illness, the Alzheimer's patient may become very stiff and rigid and exhibit symptoms that are typical of Parkinson's disease. He may lean when he walks and develop a shuffling gait. (The same symptoms may also be due to a small stroke, delirium, or the effects of medications and can in some cases be relieved. Always check with the doctor if your patient shows any change in his walk or posture.) These weaknesses can contribute to a fall, as they did in Mr. Sellers's case:

> "Last Friday morning, the home health attendant didn't show up. So I had to take my husband from the bed and walk him to the bathroom. He can't get there by himself, because his body gets very rigid, and he can only take little shuffling steps. There I was, holding on to him, helping

him to hold on to the furniture as I led him to the bathroom, when he lost his balance and fell. As he fell, he pulled me down so I fell on top of him. Luckily, neither of us was hurt; but I couldn't pick him up, so I had to call my next-door neighbor, who is a big man, to help me get Bart back to bed. He wasn't badly hurt, but the fright! He got very upset. I was so upset, too—I was just trembling. Later, I looked him over for cuts and bruises; he seemed to be okay."

Mrs. Sellers wisely inspected her husband for injuries. Because the patient may not be able to tell us he is in pain, routine checks of his body should be made.

To help him walk in future situations, Mrs. Sellers, instead of helping him hold on to furniture, should ask him to take her arm. If railings were installed in the hall at hand-height, her husband could lean on them while she steadied him from behind by holding onto his belt. Walking behind him would avoid the risk of her being thrown off balance or knocked over if he should stumble.

Mr. Sellers may still be able to learn to use a walker or a cane. Or Mrs. Sellers could ask a physical therapist to suggest other ways in which she could help her husband without hurting herself.

If your relative falls, try to stay calm. Check for any conspicuous injuries, signs of pain or bruises, swelling, or agitation. If he has hit his head, call the doctor at once; if not, reassure him and, if possible, let him get up, slowly, under his own power.

STRUCTURING THE ENVIRONMENT

If someone shows us a way to improve a skill, such as a new cooking technique, we have the option of trying it and deciding whether or not to adopt it. The person with Alzheimer's or another memory-impairing disease has no such option. He has lost his ability to learn new information.

Sometimes this loss is revealed by a change in environment, such as a move to a retirement home, or even an overnight trip. Don James travelled with his father to the funeral of an uncle two years ago. They stayed overnight and shared a room in a hotel there.

"In the middle of the night I heard a noise and was aware that Dad had gotten out of bed. Then I heard the door slam and I suddenly realized that he'd gone out in the hall.

"I went out to find out what had happened, and there he was, wandering up and down the hall, saying 'Where am I? What am I doing here?'

"Since then, we've discovered that he gets lost everywhere except at home. Mother has reorganized the house so that he has fewer choices to make. She put his bed against a wall. He can only get out of it on one side, so he always takes the same path to the bathroom. He gets along better in a very organized environment."

It is helpful to the patient to do as Mrs. James has done—to use existing and remembered habits when possible and to limit the number of options. Although the memory of even the longest-held habits will also diminish in time, during the early stages of the illness a patient living in a familiar and regulated environment is generally able to be more self-sufficient. Not only will he be less confused and disoriented, but you will find life easier when there is a sense of order in your house.

Ms. Fiermosca: "My house is very well organized. We have a wall calendar, a wall clock, and a chart of activities that my mother keeps. Mother is still physically active but terribly forgetful. She helps around the house as much as she can. She fills the food and water dishes for the dog and the parakeet, and she makes the beds every morning. We keep a chart for each job, and on it we mark off when she completes an activity. On another chart we mark off when each animal has been fed. It makes Mom feel useful.

"I have found that this structure helps her and helps me. Instead of her getting up in the morning and repeating 'What day is it? What day is it? What day is it?' we go over to the calendar and check it off. She keeps running back to the calendar when she forgets the day or the date."

You can reduce the amount of confusion your relative experiences by organizing his room and his possessions and by labeling objects that he regularly uses.

> Ms. Filmore: "I'm well organized, and it does help. When my parents died, Aunt Betty inherited the big old family home and invited my family and me to move in with her. She was becoming disoriented, and soon after we arrived it became clear that she was deteriorating rapidly. So my husband and I called in a carpenter and set up an entire suite in the house for her. Everything she owned we put right there at her fingertips so she didn't have to wander all over the house looking for her things. She has a closet, dresser, bedside table, lamp, and desk in her own room."

Ms. Filmore is fortunate that Aunt Betty has been able to adapt to the changes in her environment. The patient's inability to remember a new room or furniture arrangement may cause his family some embarrassment. A spouse, son, or daughter can be mortified by a mother who walks naked into the hotel corridor or a husband who opens the hall closet and urinates into it. When incidents like these occur, it is difficult to refrain from lashing out at the relative. A sarcastic "What did you do that for?" is useless—your relative doesn't know, can't say, and is probably embarrassed as well. Your verbal attack may make him angry and frustrated in turn.

Ms. Filmore's methods of helping her aunt feel at home in her own surroundings have been used by many caregivers. Especially in cases of mild memory impairment and in the early stages of Alzheimer's disease, labels, pictures, notes, and reminders of all sorts help the patient to maintain his confidence and independence. If he enjoys helping in the kitchen, you can label silverware drawers and cabinets where dishes are kept. Put pictures of stored objects on their cabinets (a drawing of a broom on the broom closet, for example).

If your relative was always orderly and methodical, that personality pattern is likely to persist. In such a case, you and the impaired person can make lists together, to remind him of tasks to do or the names of people he sees frequently. But don't expect a person who was never a list maker to become one now. Imposing such a new demand on your relative will probably frustrate and upset both of you.

You can help your impaired family member to recall everyday facts such as the day, the date, and the city he lives in. Mr. Chisolm has learned the best way to proceed:

> "I used to ask my sister, 'What day is it?'" and so on, every morning. I don't ask any more, and I'll tell you why. I had dinner with an old friend of mine a few days ago. He knows a thing or two about my sister's condition because he had a sister-in-law who also was affected. He told me that it really doesn't do any good to ask my sister what day it is, or what her name is. Furthermore, he told me it isn't very kind to her. 'How would you feel,' he asked me, 'if I demanded that you tell me, every day, the basic principles of nuclear physics? That would be as difficult for you as remembering the date may be for her.'
>
> "When I thought about it that way, I realized that I would be very frustrated, and I might get annoyed or upset. 'Instead of asking the questions,' he said, 'give her the answers: "Today is the 27th of April; it's Thursday; you are my sister, your name is Maryanne," and so on.'
>
> "That's what I've been doing this week, and maybe she's a little less agitated and upset. I've been trying to put myself in my sister's shoes and that helps me to be more understanding of her."

A structured environment makes life more comfortable for you and your relative, but, unfortunately, orderliness is often difficult to maintain. As a result of his disability, the forgetful person is likely to disorder things as quickly as you organize them.

> Ms. JOHNSTON: "My father is going to drive me up the wall. He takes all his tools from the tool bench and hides them all over the house. The other day, I opened the desk drawer and found a pipe wrench there. He hides my tools, too—he's taken the can opener, and I can't find it anywhere. He's so stubborn, he refuses to put things where they belong."
>
> Ms. SCHULMAN: "I came home exhausted from a business trip to discover that mother had completely upset our apartment. I couldn't find

anything: knives, forks, dishes, pots, and pans were all disarranged. All the chairs were turned around and out of place.

"I was stunned and disbelieving and hysterical, all at once. It felt as if someone had come in and ransacked the place. It seemed that she had let go with a kind of destructiveness that was aimed at me. I started screaming and yelling. I thought I would go out of my mind with the confusion she created!"

It is difficult to accept the fact that a relative is no longer capable of the simple ordinary business of living that he has carried on for a life-time, that he can no longer dress himself or put things away in their proper places. We would rather deny that anything is wrong with his brain and ascribe his behavior to willful destructiveness (as Ms. Schulman did in describing her mother's actions) or obstinacy (which Ms. Johnson believed was motivating her father).

At the same time, the disarray itself intensifies our feelings of help-lessness. Even so, an angry response, however understandable, may serve to confuse and upset your patient even further.

There is no simple solution, no single way to cope with the mess and disorder that a confused person can create. Mr. Fox has found a solution that is comfortable for him, although it may not work for everyone.

"I follow my wife wherever she goes, and I put back the things that she strews around, because she constantly takes things out and puts them down and moves them out of place. I put her clothes and shoes away, and I straighten the lamp and everything else. I do all these things in self-defense, so that I have an environment I can live in!"

The Consequences of Forgetfulness

Many problems encountered by the patient with Alzheimer's disease and his family relate to the loss of recent memory. When your relative repeats the same question again and again, fails to give you an important telephone message, can't remember where he spent the twenty dollars you gave him yesterday, or doesn't know when it's noon and time for lunch, it's distressing and can make you lose patience. Especially when the family is forced to change long-held roles, such as who drives the car and who pays the bills, the added responsibilities, combined with all the other changes in your life, can be very burdensome. Many daily problems involve the reduction of your patient's independence. These situations are difficult for you and painful for your loved one.

Perhaps our experience and that of other caregivers like yourself will help to explain some of these behaviors and give you some ideas for coping with them, and for understanding and managing your own emotional reactions as well.

DRIVING THE CAR

An illness such as Alzheimer's disease can force restriction of the patient's activity for safety reasons. For example, when it becomes necessary for your relative to stop driving the car, he may feel that much more than his ability to drive has been lost. For many people, driving the car is equated with a sense of personal freedom, of self-esteem and independence; the loss of being able to function independently can be very threatening. When a memory-impaired person can no longer go to the local store because he can't find his way home, such a restriction threatens his self-respect.

MS. JOYCE DOWNING: "One of the first serious problems we had with my father, when he developed Alzheimer's disease, was with driving. How we all survived that first year and a half I'll never know. He blamed the white lines—he said that people didn't paint those lines right. And the other drivers were all cockeyed. He insisted that he had to drive, because he was the man in the family. When he finally said, on his own, 'I have no more patience with driving,' I'm telling you, it was a relief. I didn't care if all of us were killed together—that would have been the easy way out. I was worried about what he could do to the other people on the road."

Ms. Downing illustrates the reluctance of family members to interfere with or impede the independent actions of the memory-impaired person. Memory-impaired people are a poor risk when they are confused or likely to become anxious or aggressive in traffic. They may be slow to react in an emergency or may have diminished sight or hearing. Allowing a confused person to continue to drive the family car is a source of worry to the family and can be very dangerous to the occupants of the car and to others on the road.

To preserve the patient's self-esteem and feeling of independence, some families develop elaborate sets of reasons why another person should drive each time they take a trip. These excuses may include suggestions that the impaired relative doesn't know a new route; that weather conditions may make the car hard to control; that it is "his turn" to enjoy the scenery; that he may be a little tired today. Last-ditch measures include confiscating the car keys, removing the car to a repair shop, or selling it outright. But, if you are a spouse and can drive, why not take over the driving? It will give you a feeling of competence and still allow you the freedom that an automobile can offer for marketing, visiting friends, or taking daily trips and vacations.

HANDLING MONEY AND FINANCES

In the early stages of Alzheimer's disease, a patient may be able to comprehend and even participate in decisions about money. In that case, get the family's legal and financial records together and discuss them. Allow the patient to tell you his wishes for the near future.

The memory-impaired person who has a difficult time with numbers and telling time may also have trouble with money matters. Calculating involves a complex mental process that demands the intellectual prowess of an adequately functioning brain.

MR. OSCAR BIRKLUND: "I'm very anxious about my brother, who is spending a lot of money. He's not aware of it, but he goes to the bank every day and withdraws money and spends it. He never comes home

213

with anything practical like clothes or food. I don't know where his money goes. What happens when his money is all gone—is he going to come ask me to support him? Sometimes, when I ask him about his money, he accuses me of stealing it. I don't want to be told, 'You took all of my money. Where's my money?' His accusations are terrible. He makes me feel like a thief."

Being unable to give the right amount of change to a storekeeper or to write a check for purchases, mismanaging money, spending inordinate amounts, or accusing others of stealing money are some of the indications that the impaired person's brain is deteriorating further. If he is unable to remember what he did with his money, then it is understandable that he would be anxious and suspicious about what happened to it. Managing our own money is a symbol of independence that we have had since we received our first childhood allowance. Earning one's own way in life is a further symbol of self-sufficiency; having to give up control of the purse strings represents a loss of that independence. Therefore the issue of money may bring up very severe problems, as it did for Barbara Packer:

"My brother was a very successful businessman. He and his wife had no children, and she died some years ago. He decided to take advantage of the tax laws and help me out, so he gave me a certain sum of money every year. Then his memory began to go. He got to thinking that he shouldn't have given me that money, and he wanted it back. Well, my children told me that I shouldn't give it back, that he'd given it to me of his free will; and besides, I needed it not only for myself, but also to help take care of him.

"He became very abusive and shouted at me over the phone and threatened to come over to the house and beat me up. So I left my house and stayed with friends. And even though I have changed the locks on my doors, and he doesn't have the key, I'm afraid to go home."

Both Ms. Packer and her brother are very angry and upset. Her brother will forget the incident long before Ms. Packer. That is the nature of the illness and perhaps its only blessing—that the impaired person soon forgets his accusations and his anger.

The issue of money sometimes arouses more intense feelings that the issue of sex. We're not going to tell you what should have been, because that's not really important. We're interested in what is happening now. What are your feelings about money? Who pays the bills in your household? Do you have feelings about who controls the money? Perhaps you're worried that your money is going to be dissipated by your confused spouse.

The caregiver who is not easily shaken may be able to use some ingenuity to find a challenging solution to these difficulties. If your spouse is going to forget whether or not you take over the account, you might as well take over the account. Offer him a smaller sum of money as a way of placating him so he doesn't become enraged. He can do what he wants with it. Or you can open a charge account for him at one or two places he frequents. Be sure to establish a credit limit with the stores in advance.

You probably will have to take over your relative's checkbook and pay the bills for him. It might even be a relief to the memory-impaired person; if he asks you about it, remind him gently that you are taking care of the checkbook and he need not worry.

Ms. Elizabeth Kalb was afraid to bring up the subject of money for fear of enraging her husband. So she would empty his pants pockets after he went to the bank and leave just a few dollars for him to spend. He never seemed to miss the money she took. As he became more impaired, she took over his account and continued to stuff his pants pockets with two or three one-dollar bills, so that he wouldn't be without some cash. Gradually he lost interest in buying things and seemed to forget that money is even necessary.

PROBLEMS WITH THE TELEPHONE

MR. JIM WALLER: "When the phone rings, I don't let my Dad answer it anymore because it could be business. He can't take messages well. The person on the other end of the phone will ask, 'Where's Jim?' and I'll be standing right next to him and he'll say, 'He's not here today.'"

The telephone can become a source of upset when the memory-impaired person is left alone at home. He might answer the telephone but then forget to relay the message. Some families have missed important events because the confused person took a call and forgot its content. Your relative may also begin to make a telephone call, then forget who he is calling and why he made the call. It is easiest to avoid the "your-forgetfulness-is-driving-me-mad, why-didn't-you-tell-me-about-Jack's-call, it-was-important" scene by turning the telephone off when you leave the house. On most telephones you can adjust the bell so that it is too soft for your relative to hear. Usually telephone equipment stores carry an easily installed device to turn the telephone on or off.

Tell your friends and acquaintances when you will be available to speak with them by telephone or that you'll call them. You can also buy an automatic answering machine, which picks up telephone calls and records messages. Some of these devices also have a remote calling feature by which you can call your own phone from any distance and pick up your messages.

WANDERING AND GETTING LOST

Mrs. Maureen Cobbler noticed that her husband Fred was absent-minded, but she thought little of it until he was dismissed from his factory job for making too many mistakes on the assembly line. Once he had retired, he began to visit a senior citizen's center every day while Maureen worked. He was walking to the center and back by himself, approximately two and a half miles each way, but then he began getting lost and the police brought him home.

Maureen arranged to have the senior citizen's center bus pick Fred up, but he would wander off the front porch and the bus driver wouldn't be able to find him. So Maureen began driving Fred to the center on her way to work. The bus could take him home, because he was already at the center and couldn't get lost waiting for the bus. When he got home, a neighbor came over to let him in the house and stayed with him so he wouldn't wander off before Maureen got home.

Mrs. Cobbler would have been spared much upset and difficulty had her husband worn an identification bracelet. Fred Cobbler's wandering behavior is typical of many memory-impaired people who lose the ability to remember their surroundings. Not being able to remember either where they are going or where they've been, patients with Alzheimer's and similar diseases are likely to get lost even in their own neighborhoods.

Ms. Marie Tanner: "My husband wanders something terrible! He won't sit still; he keeps moving around. It's frenetic!

"I lost him in Macy's one day. I was standing in line to pay the cashier. He was right behind me, but when I turned around, suddenly he was gone. So I asked the clerk, 'Where is your Lost & Found?'

"She said, 'What did you lose?'

"I said, 'My husband.'

"She said, 'Have him paged.'

"I started to explain that I couldn't have him paged because of his memory problem, but while I was explaining, I heard my own name over the paging system.

"You see, several years ago, when my husband first became very forgetful, I got him an ID bracelet, with his name and address and telephone number on it and the words 'Memory Impaired.' He wears it all the time. I think it's safer than carrying an ID in his wallet, because he might lose that. Besides, if the ID were in his wallet and he got lost and the police found him, the officer would have to go through his clothes looking for identification. That might upset Fred. This way, it's immediately visible and easy to find."

Most hospital gift shops sell ID bracelets such as Mr. Tanner's. They are also available by mail from Medic Alert. The Medic Alert ID is a metal emblem, worn as a necklace or bracelet, on the back of which is engraved the wearer's member identification number and special medical condition, along with a twenty-four-hour telephone number. In a central file at that number, available to anyone who makes a collect call, is vital information such as the wearer's name, address, telephone number, nearest relative, and the family physician's name, address, and telephone number. The Medic Alert Foundation International is a charitable organization that charges a one-time membership fee.

Wearing Medic Alert identification can help to avert a tragedy or fatal mistakes in emergency treatment. It can also help you locate your relative should he wander or get lost. Because of its usefulness, caregivers and memory-impaired patients alike often wear a Medic Alert emblem. One caregiver, who has a history of heart trouble, talked his forgetful spouse into wearing an identification bracelet by promising to wear one himself. He pointed out to her that she would feel much more comfortable knowing he could get help, and that she could give him the same comfort.

A standard identification bracelet that you can buy in a jewelry store may serve the purpose. For people who resist the idea of wearing jewelry, a badge pinned to the inside of a coat or jacket with name, address, telephone number, and the words "Memory Impaired" may serve. It is easier to lose, however, if the patient removes his coat and forgets where he put it.

If your patient has a tendency to lose weight, and you fear that he might lose a bracelet in a fixed size, you might want to try the type of plastic ID bracelet used in hospitals, which can be adjusted to fit any wrist. It is waterproof and has plenty of room to write in necessary information.

Sleeplessness and Night Wandering

Patients with Alzheimer's disease often seem to become more agitated as evening falls; then behavior problems become exaggerated. Perhaps Alzheimer's disease has altered the patient's natural tendency to be active by day and subdued at night. Possibly he is reacting to disturbing dreams, or to the effects of tranquilizers. Perhaps because there is less daylight, the older person cannot see as well and becomes disoriented.

The patient who is not tired enough to sleep may become a nocturnal wanderer. When he gets up, he will dress himself and behave as if it were daytime; then he may fall asleep in a chair with all of his clothes on. It is wise to let these things pass as long as you, the caregiver, can get some sleep.

To reduce the likelihood of night wandering, see that the patient has enough activity and exercise during the day so that he will be tired at night. Make sure he uses the bathroom just before bedtime. He will then be less likely to be wakened by a full bladder.

To keep your relative safe, and to avoid his being alarmed upon awakening, leave a night-light in the bedroom, in the bathroom, and in other rooms in the house; thus, he will never awaken to total darkness. Make sure doors and windows are locked and that dangerous areas such as stairways are protected with gates. If he awakens with a start and is alarmed, try to reassure him.

If these precautions are insufficient, you and your physician may consider a sleeping pill or a major tranquilizer. To avoid the hangover effect of sedatives, start with a smaller dosage and gradually increase it until it achieves maximum effectiveness.

It is especially important that the caregiver get sufficient rest and sleep. Feeling dragged out from lack of sleep contributes to irritability and decreases your tolerance for frustration.

> MR. ROGER GOWAN: "My wife sleeps for about five solid hours. Then she'll get up, about five in the morning, and start shuffling around. I hear the toilet bowl flushing and flushing until I almost go crazy. Lillian takes toilet tissue and rolls it up in her hand, wiping her face, her neck, her head, and throwing it in the toilet and flushing it, over and over again. That can go on for hours unless I get out of bed and put a stop to it."

It is probable that, in consultation with his wife's physician, Mr. Gowan can find a sleeping pill or other medication that is safe for his wife to take and that will keep her sleeping longer than five hours a night. He seems to be able to stop her annoying behavior, once he is aware of it, without creating anger or panic on her part.

Many caregivers find that they need help in caring for and managing their afflicted relatives at home. A professional home health aide or practical nurse can relieve you of some of the daytime—or nighttime—burden of caring for your relative so you can get sufficient rest.

However, it's important to remember that even additional help cannot solve every problem. Perhaps you can devise your own creative solution to the problem of night wandering, as Mrs. Crosley did.

Rita Crosley's father-in-law came to live with her and her husband Bart ten years ago, when Bart's mother died. It was a natural move—the Crosleys have plenty of room, and Bart is the "Son" of Crosley & Son, his father's business. Things went pretty smoothly until the senior Mr. Crosley developed Alzheimer's disease five years later.

Recently, when his father could no longer handle the business properly, Bart Crosley took it over completely, But Mr. Crosley was accustomed to getting up every morning and going to the office. He had always gone to the office very early, at about 5:30 in the morning, while it was still dark during most of the year. "So," Mrs. Crosley reports, "for Dad, night is day and day is night. He's been getting up any time from midnight to dawn, and turning on all the lights and getting ready to go to work. Sometimes I think I'll go out of my mind with it."

But Mrs. Crosley has been equal to the situation and has found at least a temporary solution.

She hid the clothes that he would ordinarily wear to go to work. He gets up in the middle of the night and, seeing that his clothes aren't there, goes down the hall to the door of Bart and Rita's room and asks, "Where are my clothes?"

Then Rita says to him, "You don't see them set out for you, do you? When you don't see them set out, that means you don't have to go to work." She may have to repeat it once or twice, but eventually he grasps the idea and goes back to bed.

"In terms of getting him back to bed," she remarks, "it seems to be working. I've taken the clothes out of the drawers—there's no underwear, no socks, no shoes—nothing. If I wake up before he comes down the hall, I can hear him pulling out the empty drawers.

"But after he goes back to sleep, I'm up for the rest of the night. I can't fall asleep after that. He can get his rest, but I can't get mine."

If you, like Mrs. Crosley, have dealt with the immediate problem of getting your relative back to bed, but then find yourself awake, agitated, and unable to sleep, you might try one of the relaxation techniques developed by researchers who study sleep habits. Some are as simple as the old-fashioned counting of sheep (or any repetitive number of objects that you imagine are passing before your eyes). Many people find that meditation techniques help them to drop off to sleep. One insomniac we know has discovered the magic of a special fantasy: he found that the most difficult part of getting back to sleep was worrying about having to start the new day in just a few hours. He was able to go to sleep easily when he told himself, over and over, "You have many more hours to sleep. You can sleep and be rested for tomorrow." Perhaps a similar form of self-hypnosis will work for you.

When you are faced with night-waking behavior on the part of your impaired parent, spouse, or sibling, try to be as inventive as possible, both in getting your patient to return to bed and in making it possible for you, too, to get some rest. Many caregivers have discovered that arguing with a wakeful patient only makes him irritated, confused, and possibly even violent. As exhausted as you probably are, try to remain calm and quiet and, if possible, soothe the person back to bed. Then, when you have an opportunity to be by yourself, soothe yourself with your own relaxation techniques.

Whatever your solution, we cannot overstress your need for your own time, privacy, rest, and relaxation. It is as important as the need to pacify and calm your relative so he can return to sleep.

CHAPTER 13

The Nursing Home Dilemma

Americans tend to think of nursing homes with disgust and aversion. Although one-quarter of all elderly Americans will spend some time in a nursing home, for many the thought of living in a nursing home is associated with feelings of uselessness, loneliness, and abandonment. These feelings toward nursing homes often exist in both older and younger Americans even when the only such institutions they have seen are pleasant, airy, cheerful places. Certainly the most attractive institution, perceived through the curtain of such attitudes, can seem to be a dismal place.

Furthermore, it is difficult to be reassured by the treatment generally given to nursing homes by television and the public press. The fear that a beloved relative might suffer from mistreatment in such an environment drives many families to go to extraordinary lengths to keep an elderly impaired person at home—in his own home, if possible, or, if need be, in the home of an adult child or sibling.

Yet there are many situations in which placing a confused relative in a nursing home eases not only the patient's circumstances but the pressures on other family members as well. In some cases, the unexamined refusal to consider a nursing home for a memory-impaired relative causes more unhappiness and stress for a family than it would experience if it were to choose institutionalization. Even so, the overwhelming choice of families is to try to help the confused elder remain and function in a familiar apartment, neighborhood, or environment.

Often the ability to do this depends on emotional and economic assistance from other family members and the availability of support systems in the community. By support systems we mean arranging services for home health attendants, visiting nurse services, the delivery of meals, transportation to day care centers, and other services that the older person living at home finds essential. Physical, occupational, and speech therapy, if required, can be brought to the patient at home. Medical care and other home services can be provided in a "nursing home without walls" environment in the home of the patient. With these support systems, the advantages of home care seem obvious. When the caregiver is also able to have some recreation and respite, home care becomes the atmosphere of choice.

The caregiver who participates in the physical care of a chronically ill person by providing needed services with love and concern increases the patient's comfort and security. The patient's morale is also better in a familiar environment. Indeed, research bears this out: confused patients, who seem particularly vulnerable to the stress of sudden change, tend to deteriorate rapidly in unfamiliar surroundings.

Emily Tinknor told us about her husband Danny, who started developing Alzheimer's disease about twelve years ago. He had to quit work almost immediately. For the next half-dozen years he could handle himself, travel around the city, do the laundry and errands for her. About six years ago, Danny began to get worse. Now, he's like a child. For the last six months he hasn't been able to bathe or dress himself and he can't understand words. During the years that Danny was impaired, Emily assumed that he would die first, and that she would take care of him until the end. In the last few months, she's had to accept the fact that she might not have the physical stamina to continue caring for him. She might have to consider putting him in a nursing home. Yet Emily feels that if Danny went to a home, he would want to leave the minute he got there. She has read that people get worse in nursing homes.

There is some truth to Mrs. Tinknor's fears. Research shows that some people die within the first three months after being placed in a nursing home. Many factors account for this, including the health of the patient—terminally ill patients are often moved from hospitals to nursing homes or hospices. But when the family members continue to visit and maintain an interest in the patient, their behavior may help to mitigate the confusion caused by new people and different surroundings.

Decision-Making

Deciding to place the confused family member in a long-term care facility such as a nursing home is difficult for most families and gives rise to intense and ambivalent feelings. Each situation is unique, and the decision is usually based on the caregiver's physical and emotional resources as well as threshold of frustration tolerance. Some families are able to accept disturbing and erratic behavior and will endure great hardship to keep their relatives at home. Others, more vulnerable or with fewer coping abilities, decide at an earlier stage that an alternative to home care must be sought.

When a family decides that it is in its own and the impaired relative's best interest to seek a different residence, it should be a joint decision if the impaired person is able to participate in the decision-making process.

All too often families avoid the painful decision to put a relative in a nursing home until there is a crisis, when decisions must be made hurriedly. In moments of crisis, choices are limited. Families that decide to place a loved one in a hastily selected institution will probably suffer much guilt for not having previously investigated accommodations for their impaired relative.

Caregivers have experienced finding a suitable nursing home as a long and difficult process; they have also heard distressing stories of nursing home abuses; or they have had previous upsetting experiences with an institutionalized friend or relative. While they wrestle with their own ambivalent feelings, they are aware of the need to have some personal respite and a reprieve from the constant caregiving. But the pangs of conscience produce, at the same time, guilty feelings about making such a decision to lighten their burden.

MRS. PRENTISS: "My husband is treated by his own doctor, but my nephew, who is an internist, takes care of me. My husband's doctor prescribed a tranquilizer for him because he was very agitated, but the dosage was too large, so he became zombielike. Of course we reduced the dosage immediately, but even so, my nephew was shocked when he saw my husband. He said, 'He's under a drug, too doped—they do that in nursing homes!' It made a deep impression on me. If that's what a doctor thinks of nursing homes, how can I consider putting my husband there?"

MS. BRIDGES: "In the nursing home, it isn't the doctor or the nurse that handles most of my sister's needs. It's an aide that comes in, for example, to feed her.

"I get so frustrated and angry when I see some insensitive young thing, who knows nothing, yelling at my sister because my sister is not eating, or because she's playing with her food. The aide wants to shove the food into my poor sister's mouth. My sister can't protest because she's lost her voice—she can't talk any more. Maybe her mouth can't move fast enough, or there's some other problem. But this aide has the responsibility of feeding my sister, and she's not kind to my sister. This is a terrible thing!

"There should be a program in these institutions so that someone who is trained in dealing with these victims and knows how to care for them is assigned to them."

Stories like those of Mrs. Prentiss and Ms. Bridges can deter a caregiver from carrying out a decision to institutionalize a relative. The nursing home scandals that have been reported in the media have given the public a very negative image of nursing homes, much like the image of the "snake pit" for the mentally disturbed of yesteryear. Nursing homes are thought to be dirty, smelly places where residents are intimidated or abused by the staff, the food is of the lowest quality, and people are warehoused and left to die. We know that there are good nursing homes, less satisfactory ones, and even today, some that we would like to put out of business. However, present-day nursing home abuses, fortunately, have been reduced or largely eliminated. Every state has strict regulations by which nursing homes must abide, and inspections are made on a regular basis. There is a Resident's Bill of Rights (see Appendix B), and nursing homes are subject to severe censure if the rights of a resident are violated.

It is a regrettable fact that fear of retaliation against the patient may keep him or his family from reporting an abuse. Families fear that the patient will be sent home from the institution if they report an abuse, and that fear may keep them from making a complaint to the nursing home administrator. In fact, the reverse is true: patients' and families' complaints actually ensure that the patient will get better care. It is the timid resident, who is afraid to speak up and has no one to be his advocate, who is more likely to be a victim.

Some nursing homes have ombudspersons who protect the rights of the apparently helpless residents. Others have organized family support groups for the relatives of residents.

AMBIVALENT FEELINGS

MR. GALLAGHER: "There are many times when I say I wish it were over. You know you face the inevitable. And you say, 'Why go through this torture for her and for yourself? It would be kinder if it were quicker, both for her and for you.'

"My son-in-law is trying to pressure me into putting her in a nursing home.

"I'm very ambivalent about that. There are days when things are quieter, and better, and I say, 'Why do it? We'll cope!' And then there are days when I can't wait to get her in. There are days when she's more amenable to suggestion, at which point I say, 'Of course, we'll go on this way.' But lately she is becoming incontinent, and I have to supervise her when she goes to the bathroom to make sure that she sits down properly. Otherwise there might be an accident. It's getting to where I feel very distressed by the whole situation. And the pain of watching her deteriorate is keeping me up nights.

"Since I know that this is just the beginning, and that it won't improve, I'm considering putting her into a nursing home.

"I wonder if I'm doing the right thing to put her in an institution . . . I look at what's going on in these places, at people strapped to chairs, held in restraints, or tied, and when I think that eventually this might be my own wife, it scares me. Yet the children keep saying, 'Do it Dad. What if something happened to you, Dad?'

"In fact, even as I'm looking at nursing homes and putting her name on waiting lists, I'm telling myself that perhaps I can get someone for the nights and keep her at home. I have such ambivalence about the whole question."

An elderly caregiver, Mrs. Cobb, fears that she will die before her husband, so that her children will have the burden of caring for him. "I would like to outlive my husband by maybe just one day. That's all I ask."

And Mr. Kolb's children think he should be considering a nursing home for his wife Marie. Because he's a spouse, and not a child, he would have to pay full fee for as long as he was able. The cost would come to forty or fifty thousand dollars a year. Mr. Kolb's lawyer tried to show him how he could manage it. Finally, the lawyer suggested that he talk to his accountant.

Both the lawyer and the accountant have relatives of their own in nursing homes, so they have firsthand knowledge. When Mr. Kolb called the accountant and told him what the lawyer had said about Marie, the accountant said, "Look—she's ambulatory, she likes to walk, she's continent, she can eat without help, and she always looks very well dressed and well groomed—why don't you wait? What's your hurry? The day she becomes incontinent . . . ."

Mr. Kolb is right back where he was, with pressures both for and against placing his wife in a nursing home. Marie loves to walk and goes out every day. But if someone's not with her, she has a tendency to wander away. So either he would have to hire a companion for her in the nursing home, which is over and above and basic fee, or he would have to consent to having her strapped in—as he says, like a domestic animal.

THE SPECIAL CONCERNS OF ADULT CHILDREN

Children who are faced with the need to put one or both of their parents into a nursing home often feel very guilty, as if they didn't love their parents enough. Some parents think that children should feel guilty if they don't take care of their parents. After raising the children to adulthood, there are parents who expect their children to feel a sense of responsibility for the lives of their elderly parents. While some children do agree with this viewpoint, those who do not may be a great disappointment to their parents.

Mrs. Ortiz sees her husband every day. His case was a rapidly progressing one. He's only 60 years old, and although he has only had the disease for a year, he's already in a nursing home. He can't talk, and he must be fed. Every day Mrs. Ortiz tries to visit the nursing home in time to feed Mr. Ortiz his dinner. Seeing him every day sustains her.

But their children don't see him anymore. During the first week that he was in the institution, they visited, a few times each. Since then, they've told her that they can't stand to see him any more. They say it's such a shock to see what has happened to this very beautiful person, both inwardly and outwardly, that they get too upset when they see him.

At a certain level, Mrs. Ortiz can understand the way her children feel. But underneath, she really resents them. She cannot believe that her child would just say "I can't see him any more" and stay away. It is difficult to accept their not seeing him again. She feels she could never have behaved that way to her parents.

Ms. Tremaine: "I love my mother, but I resent the responsibility of caring for her. It's really all-consuming, especially when you are, as I am, an only child. I get very angry with her, and then I feel so guilty. I can't do anything for my own family, or for myself.

"You're supposed to take care of your mother. That was drummed into me when I was a child. My mother told me over and over that my father said to her how lucky she was to have a girl, because a girl-child would take care of her when she was old. I think it's wrong. I would never teach that to my own children.

"Mother was in her forties when I was born. When I was younger, I swore that I would always take care of her. I never actually believed it would happen; she was such a self-sufficient woman. Now, she's totally dependent, and the responsibility is so overwhelming that I can't handle it.

"I'm afraid she just won't wake up one day. I even sell my children short to tend to her, because each day may be her last day. Part of me realizes that she could still live for several more years.

"I kept her out of a nursing home as long as I could. Now that she's there, I visit her almost daily. I think it's a good idea to go often, since I'm the one that represents the family. Even when I don't visit her, I don't seem to be able to do my housekeeping properly. I'm depressed and I feel guilty that she's in the nursing home. I don't feel that I'm doing all that I should for her, because I'm not physically taking care of her. But when she was with me in my home, everything was a mess. I would get very angry at her when she lost control of her bowels and soiled herself.

"Caring for anyone who's senile is a very, very big job if you take it seriously. I consider it to be a full-time job and if you are the only person doing it, it's too much of a responsibility and a burden. How much can one person carry?"

The experience of putting a feeble and confused parent into a nursing home can change the way we view parent-child relationships, and our attitudes toward our own eventual aging:

MR. GRESHAM: "I don't want my children to have to live through this guilt that I'm living with, and this ambivalence toward my father. I want to do everything for him, but I don't know what 'everything' is, and I certainly don't have time to do everything.

"I intend to tell the kids in a very logical, reasonable way that when the time comes that I cannot take care of myself, I want them to use all their ingenuity to find me the best possible place available at that moment; I mean a nursing home. I want them to have that much responsibility. But I want to tell them now, at this point, while they're still young and reasonable, that I don't want them to feel they have to take care of me, directly, physically, in their own homes. And I'll tell them that if I say anything later to the opposite, that's not me, really. 'These are my thoughts and I'm a reasonable person. I think you would be a fine child if you would just deal with it this way.' I want to alleviate some of the guilt, if I can."

Loving families often feel torn between grief and sadness at the continual deterioration of a loved one, angry at the paucity of choices that are available to them, and guilty over their wish for someone else to assume the tremendous burden of care. Often these are feelings of having failed or abandoned a loved one in committing him to a nursing home. When the decision is finally made, the family usually experiences all these mixed feelings along with a sense of relief (which may, in turn, provoke more guilt). Sometimes the decision is precipitated by a "last straw" experience, usually when the impaired person loses control of bowel functions, as Ms. Tremaine's mother did.

It is clearly appropriate to institutionalize a person who has severe organic brain dysfunction. The criteria that are generally used to determine whether a patient is a candidate for a nursing home are that he (1) is a danger to himself and other, (2) exhibits wandering behavior, incontinence, and soiling, and (3) severely interferes with the sleep of the caregiver. When the impaired person's behavior does not respond to medication, or when he is hallucinating or suffering delusions and no longer knows who he is, institutionalization should be considered as a viable alternative to home care. Alzheimer's disease accounts for half of all elderly patients in nursing homes.

AN ACT OF LOVE

There are times when placing a relative in a nursing home is in fact an act of love. That may seem like paradoxical thinking, but consider Brenda Charles's experience.

"I love my older sister. She raised me from the time I was very small, she helped pay my way through college, and I'm enormously grateful to her. But I couldn't keep her in my house anymore. We had to send her to a nursing home.

"My sister would be better off if she weren't in the home, I think. There's nothing to recommend nursing homes. If you were to insist that loving someone means doing everything that you can for that person, then I feel I am less loving than I should be to my sister because I put her in a home instead of caring for her myself.

"But there's a balance involved. If the only person you want to consider is the patient, you can set her up in her little kingdom, and focus all your attention on her. But there are other people involved. There's the caregiver—that's me. There are my children. And the children were suffering—they weren't suffering because of Auntie Annie, nor did they mind having her there—they were suffering because of what my sister was doing to me. And the same was true of my husband. So when I weigh all those needs on a scale against Annie's increasing physical dependence and deteriorating condition, I leave her in the nursing home, although I visit her nearly every day. I could bring her back to my house, physically; I could do it, but I won't."

Ms. Charles feels guilty about putting Annie in a nursing home, but she also want to be able to attend to her husband and children. While she loves Annie, she resents her need for constant attention.

In choosing to place Annie in a nursing home, Ms. Charles did what all family members must do: she considered every aspect of her family's situation thoroughly and realistically. She used her intelligence, and at the same time she took into account the emotions involved—how she would feel about her decision. Discussing her feelings with a psychotherapist helped her to come to terms with her guilt and sadness.

A teenager told us this story:

"When I discovered that my parents had arranged for my grandmother to live in a nursing home, I deeply resented their decision. I felt angry that they were treating her like a helpless old woman. To me, she had always seemed perfect in all respects. Her beautiful garden was the result of her own meticulous care and planning. She knitted sweaters for me in

231

bright colors and trimmed them with hand-embroidered flowers. Every year on my birthday I would receive a perfect, golden pineapple upside-down cake. Her constant attention always made me feel special. I could not understand how such a creative and gifted woman could be confined to an 'old age' home.

"I didn't visit my grandmother until a month after she had been admitted into the nursing home. When I entered her room, she glanced up and smiled. It seemed that she was finally recovering from the death of my grandfather, for she had rarely smiled after he died. While we were talking, it also became clear to me that her memory had improved. Since my grandfather's death, she had been quite absentminded and could scarcely remember anyone's name.

"As I reflect upon the period before my grandmother's admittance into the nursing home, I realize that when my grandfather died, she lost all of the support that he had provided. Although she still has some problems with memory, and sometimes gets confused and thinks that the nursing home is a country club, the security that she is now receiving from the nursing home has helped her overcome her feelings of fear and depression."

Caring family members may experience a grief reaction when they place their relative in a nursing home. It is as if the person had already died. This may be a more traumatic experience than the actual death later on. Mr. Ortiz's children typify family members who are unable to tolerate their own grief and ambivalent feelings and who therefore may stop visiting.

However, when family members maintain their involvement with the patient and visit frequently, the continuity of the relationship with the patient can help him avoid the feeling of depersonalization that is some-times experienced in an institution. Befriending staff members, bringing them information about memory impairment, and perceiving them as human beings who have a very difficult job will help you maintain good relationships for yourself and your institutionalized relative. Families may visit often, take their relatives on outings, and become involved in the life of the institution; in doing so, they assist in helping their relative make a better adjustment to the nursing home.

As you confront the question of whether or not to put your memory-impaired relative in a nursing home, we hope that you have learned to act with due caution, and with a considerable amount of forethought. Placement in an institution, whether it's for a temporary stay or a permanent one, requires careful investigation. It also requires that you examine your own feelings very thoroughly. You can consult both books and people to learn what to look for, but you must come to terms with and live with your own decision.

In the balance of this chapter, we will suggest some criteria that are useful in evaluating the nursing homes you visit and ways to make your relative's relocation to a new home as comfortable as possible.

Evaluating Patients for Nursing Home Care

Nursing homes have their own way of evaluating the level of care needed by a resident. The level-of-care rating establishes what services are necessary for the care of a patient, and a board periodically reviews all nursing home patients. In New York State, this evaluation is generally reported on a DMS form (it may have a different title in other states) that is filled out by your own physician after a recent medical examination. (In some states, nurses from visiting nurse services may also fill out the DMS form.) A recent chest X-ray is also necessary to indicate that the patient does not have tuberculosis.

The patient will be assigned to a bed on the basis of the level-of-care rating. The level-of-care rating can also determine Medicare and Medicaid eligibility, payment level, and into what kind of nursing home the person should be placed. Once you know the level-of-care rating, you will know what kind of nursing home to search for.

Shopping for a Good Nursing Home

How can you evaluate a long-term care facility into which you will put someone you love or perhaps—one day—yourself? There are questions that should be asked, the answers to which you have a right to know. But be aware that detailed inquiries are often not welcomed by institutions; further, some institutions will not allow lengthy undisturbed visits by outsiders.

You should be able to inspect the physical facilities, find out about the types of medical and nursing services available, and investigate the types of personal and social services, administration, and staff. If you are not allowed to do this or speak to the residents, or you cannot get an exact itemization of costs in a given nursing home, forget that home and go on to the next. Learn to answer your own questions through personal observation when possible; but when in doubt, ask the administrator and/or members of the staff.

When you go shopping for a nursing home, have a list of several names. It is best to get the names from families who have already placed a relative; from a gerontologist, social worker, or physician who is knowledgeable about nursing homes; or from the Department of Aging, Department of Health, County Medical Society; or, if need be, the yellow pages of a telephone directory.

Ask pointed questions when you telephone the homes you are planning to visit. Are there beds available at the level-of-care rating your relative needs? Is there a waiting list—how long? Does the home accept your funding sources? Don't ask on the phone if the home accepts patients with Alzheimer's disease. Provided that your relative meets the eligibility requirements, in theory a home cannot turn down a patient who has Alzheimer's disease. In practice, many homes do turn away these patients by stating there is no bed available for the patient (even if there is). A nursing home whose staff is not equipped to deal with a memory-impaired patient may, for that reason, turn the patient away. Don't get discouraged or feel slighted—you don't want that home anyway. You *do* want a nursing home where staff members are trained in behavior modification and can toilet-train an incontinent person. You are also looking for trained personnel whose general knowledge and abilities are such that they will react promptly, without panic or injury to the patient, if he should wander or overreact to a benign situation with a violent outburst.

ACCREDITATION AND LICENSING

Two national organizations provide objective ratings that can help you to evaluate the nursing homes you visit. The Long-Term Care Council of the Joint Commission on Accreditation of Hospitals conducts on-site reviews of the nursing home's facilities and operation to reinforce compliance with the commission's standards. This accreditation, which applies to institutions that offer skilled nursing care, should be publicly displayed. If it is not, ask the nursing home if it has been accredited by the Joint Commission. The American Health Care Association, an association of private, profit-making institutions, and its state affiliates provide peer review in which the members rate one another to maintain uniform standards. These two professional review systems ensure the quality of care you may expect for your relative in a nursing home.

Other licensing approvals to look for are memberships in a state nursing home association, the American Association of Homes for the Aging (an association of nonprofit homes), and/or the American Nursing Home Association, and a nursing home administrator license.

The most important and most easily evaluated aspect of a nursing home is licensing by proper state authorities; these licenses should be openly displayed. Licensing codes prescribe requirements for fire safety, adequate nutrition, type of staff, and the number of people necessary to attend to patients.

There are three important areas to discuss with the nursing home administrator of every home you visit. These are accreditation, financial procedures, and the quality of care for residents. Of these, the only one you can obtain in writing is a copy of the financial arrangements, specifying costs that are included in the basic charge and those that are extra. Sometimes there is an additional charge for medications, special nursing procedures, incontinence pads, laundry, beauty parlor, and aides to help the patient exercise.

Make sure the nursing home is certified to accept Medicare or Medicaid and that the home will continue to keep a privately paying patient who is then switched to Medicaid.

If the home meets your criteria for licensing and location, look into safety considerations. There should be regular fire drills, good lighting, and handrails and grab bars in bathrooms and hallways. There should be no scatter rugs, easily tipped chairs, or obstructions in corridors. Stairways should be kept closed.

Then consider food services. There should be a licensed dietician in charge of the kitchen. Ask if special diets (salt-free or kosher, for example) can be obtained and if food preferences of the patient are followed. Inspect the kitchen for cleanliness.

See if the dining rooms are cheerful and if there is room for wheelchairs at the tables. Ask if between-meal and bedtime snacks are available, and how bedridden patients are fed if they can't eat by themselves. If your visit coincides with the end of a meal, look to see if trays containing uneaten food are swiftly removed.

How comfortable a resident will feel in a nursing home depends on several factors. If city noises are something a resident has been used to for sixty years or more, the silence of the country can be unnerving. A home should be located conveniently for family members to visit, close to public transportation, and in an area where visitors will feel fairly safe. Outdoor patio areas and/or lawns for the residents' use are important. Railings in hallways and wide doorways for wheelchairs are equally important. Ideally, rooms should not be shared by more than two residents so that residents may feel some sense of privacy and can add personal touches to make the rooms more cheerful. The resident may be allowed to bring some of his own furniture if there is space. Personal and familiar objects should be brought with him. Notice whether there is a secure place or locked drawer or closet for valuables. Often there is a separate dining area accessible to patients with walkers and wheelchairs. Most nursing homes have a chapel or a peaceful area that residents can use and rooms where the public can socialize with visitors. When you visit a home, notice if such rooms are in use.

Group activities are offered in most nursing homes with a varied program of educational classes, musical events, and hobbies. There is usually a library and an entertainment center. Aides transport wheelchair patients to activities.

Group activities are important for many nursing home residents, but some, who have been solitary people most of their lives, may continue to want to keep to themselves. If that has been their lifestyle and they seem comfortable with it, it is an intrusion to insist that they attend group activities. Reading a book, listening to the radio, watching television, or talking to a responsive aide or to one visitor may be enough sociability for these people. The nursing home staff should respect the solitude of a resident and his privacy as well.

MEDICAL AND OTHER SERVICES

Your patient will need the same medical services in the nursing home that he requires in your own home. The institution you choose should have a qualified medical director who has been educated in geriatric medicine. While a resident of the home, a patient should be able to see his own private physician, although staff doctors are usually available on twenty-four hour call if necessary. For emergencies, the nursing home should have an affiliation with a nearby hospital. If your relative were to become suddenly and seriously ill, you ought to know where he would be taken.

Other forms of medical care are important too, and in your questions to the administrators of the home you will probably want to ask whether a psychiatrist, podiatrist, optometrist or ophthalmologist, and dentist are regularly available, and how often they visit. Determine, if you can, where and how medical records are kept for each patient.

Nursing care is as important, in many circumstances, as the care of a physician. To assure yourself of this aspect of patient care, find out if a registered nurse is always on duty. Besides the presence of a registered nurse, there should be enough licensed practical nurses for the number of residents. Nurses' aides and assistants should get in-service education and training.

A professional social worker who can help with admission procedures and explore alternatives to institutionalization is an asset to a nursing home and to the family contemplating placement of a memory-impaired relative there. Ideally, a social worker, psychologist, or professionally trained gerontologist should be available to help the patient and the family with personal problems, to assist in the adjustment to the nursing home, to consult with the staff about the psychological and social needs of the patient, and to discuss choices of roommates and table companions. It is lamentable that most social workers in nursing homes are inundated with paperwork. They spend most of their time filling out forms, rather than utilizing their training to be available to deal with the emotional needs of residents and their families.

Sometimes social workers will be very helpful and will take time to listen to and allay your fears and anxieties. If not, help is available on the outside—don't hesitate to ask for such help. Psychologists or psychotherapists are rarely found in nursing homes. A gerontologist is a new breed of professional who is usually only consulted privately or through a geriatric clinic or a geriatric ward in a hospital. We hope they will become a regular part of the staff of nursing homes in the future.

Rehabilitation services such as speech therapy, occupational, remotivation, and recreational therapy, and training in reality orientation and bladder control may be necessary for some patients, while physiotherapy is needed for others. All of these services should be available on a regular basis.

Services should be visible. Nursing homes, like vacation resorts, often send beautiful brochures with pictures and testimonials about the breadth of services they offer. The question is whether or not these professional services do in fact exist and whether a visitor can see them in action. You will want to see that these services make a difference and have an impact on the residents.

When you visit the home, observe whether there is a bustle of activity when you come in. A nursing home that uses large doses of medication to keep its residents peaceful, or one that keeps them in restraints instead of encouraging them to be physically active and involved, whether in exercise, physical therapy, occupational therapy, or other activities, is a home that should be ruled out.

Interaction between staff and patients should reflect concern, friendliness, and warmth. The dignity of the patient should at all times be up-held. (This is often reflected in the staff's practice of referring to all patients by their surnames.)

> MR. BLANKENBRACE: "It's terribly important that the aides treat the residents with respect. I once heard one of the staff people at the nursing home say to my father, 'Oh, you naughty boy! Why did you wet your pants?' as she was changing him.
>
> "I was furious! He's not a naughty boy—he's a grown man with a problem. I can tell by the look on his face whenever he becomes incontinent that he's mortified because he can't control his body. The last thing he needs is a scolding. He's still an adult, even though the Alzheimer's disease sometimes makes him act in childish ways. He needs to be reassured, not punished. His dignity should be bolstered, not further taken away."

In the nursing home, a person's individuality and privacy need to be respected. There must also be room for some personal freedom, al-though the very nature of institutional life means that some individual liberties must be curtailed. Conforming to the routine of a nursing home means, in and of itself, capitulation to rules, regulations, and standards made by other people. It also represents, symbolically, the loss of inde-pendence on which most elderly people pride themselves. While self-reliance and self-sufficiency have less value in a nursing home than con-formity and compliance, the dependency needs of the frail and impaired elderly person can be met in such an atmosphere.

One of the most positive aspects of a nursing home's structure is provision for a family organization that holds regular family meetings where issues are discussed that can later be brought to the attention of the administrator and/or department heads.

Another reassuring factor is the presence of a resident council that has similar access to "important people" who would improve or eliminate harmful or unlivable situations. The home should display and adhere to the Resident's Bill of Rights.

Nursing Home Care Costs

The costs of nursing home care vary from state to state, city to city, country to country, and institution to institution. They also differ in terms of sponsorship—that is, whether the homes are (a) voluntary nursing homes, which are nonprofit, religious (sectarian or nonsectarian), and managed by the laity; (b) proprietary nursing homes, which are profit-making and privately owned and managed, or (c) public nursing homes, of which there are but a handful. The American Association of Homes for the Aging, located in Washington, DC, publishes a directory of accredited voluntary homes listed by state.

The federal government formerly categorized nursing homes as either "skilled nursing homes" or "extended care facilities." Under the government's new classification, a skilled nursing facility (SNF) is one in which intensive medical and nursing care can be obtained on an extended care basis. Skilled nursing facilities are eligible for both Medicare and Medicaid.

Also created was a new category, intermediate-care facilities (ICFs), also know as health-related facilities (HRFs), which are intended to serve elderly people needing long-term residential care with medical supervision. HRFs are not equipped to provide continuous nursing supervision or special rehabilitative therapies and are reimbursed only by Medicaid.

In essence, the HRF replaces the traditional "homes for the aged" into which fairly healthy old people who needed some supervision had been placed previously.

The skilled nursing facility replaces the older concept of the convalescent home. Some SNFs also have one or more HRF floors for the less dependent older person.

Economic considerations play a substantial role in the selection of a nursing home, as they do in our choice of life-style and the quality of health care that we can purchase. There are elderly people whose income level is such that they may be able to pay the full cost of nursing home care from their own income, savings, or a private insurance policy that contributes to the cost. A veteran of the armed services may be eligible for nursing home care in a Veterans Administration facility. The U.S. government's Medicare program may contribute to the cost of caring for an elderly patient in a nursing home for a limited time, but it does *not* pay for long-term care (over 100 days). The Medicaid program, in contract, takes over the cost of the nursing home once a patient has divested himself of practically everything he has accumulated financially; it does not benefit the 95 percent of elderly people who are not in nursing homes.

The cost of nursing home care can run between $25,000 and $60,000 per year, depending on the region of the country and the quality of care. If a patient suffers a catastrophic illness, a couple's entire life savings can be spent in just thirteen weeks. A few insurance companies now offer long-term health care policies, some of which cover care in the home as well. Of course, you must buy such a policy when you are still healthy, and the cost is usually high.

More and more financial responsibility will be placed on elderly people and their families as state and federal budgets eliminate social programs, creating a double tragedy: catastrophic illness and bankruptcy. *How to Protect Your Life Savings from Catastrophic Illness and Nursing Homes,* by attorney Harley Gordon, gives valuable advice about this crisis of long-term care.

Medicare and Medicaid Explained

People often confuse the two types of aid. Not only do the two words sound somewhat alike, but the tangle of regulations governing each program seems impenetrable. The major difference is that Medicare is a *federal health insurance* program for the elderly and for some younger people who are physically disabled. Medicaid is a *federal assistance* program administered on a state level by the Social Security Administration and is available to the financially needy of all ages if they meet the eligibility requirements.

Both programs are part of the Social Security Act. An individual may be eligible for both. The following description of each program as it applies to the elderly (and to the memory-impaired patient in particular) is based on current regulations as of mid-1992. Regulations do change, so it's important that you consult a social worker in your Social Security office or someone knowledgeable about these programs to help you use them precisely to meet your individual situation.

MEDICARE

You must apply for Medicare. If you are 65 or over and have applied for and are receiving Social Security benefits, you will automatically be eligible. Three or four months after your sixty-fifth birthday, you will receive a notice and a card. (Medicare, although originally intended for the elderly, also covers people who are totally and permanently disabled and those who require kidney dialysis.)

To apply for Medicare, you must be a U.S. citizen and have resided in the United States for five years. You must also be entitled to payments under the Social Security Act or Railroad Retirement Act. You are *eligible* for Medicare when you meet the eligibility requirements. After you apply and are accepted, you become *entitled* to benefits. Medicare has two parts, A and B.

Part A—Hospital Insurance pays for inpatient hospital care and post-operative care in a skilled nursing home for up to 100 days. A limited amount of at-home convalescent care is covered under certain circumstances.

Part A is for those:

- who are age 65 or over and are eligible for Social Security or Railroad Retirement;
- who are of any age and have received Social Security Disability for twenty-four months;
- who reached the age of 65 before 1974 but are not eligible for Social Security.

People 65 and over who are not eligible for Social Security can get Part A of Medicare by paying a premium for the coverage; thus, even a millionaire could receive Medicare.

At the beginning of a hospitalization, the patient must pay $628 (as of 1991), which is the deductible. Medicare should then pay all of the hospital charges for the first sixty days, as well as hospital and laboratory tests. Private rooms or television, telephone, and private duty nurses are not covered. If the patient must remain in the hospital for more than sixty days, he must pay $157 a day for the sixty-first to the ninetieth day and $314 for any additional days. Medicare pays the rest. If, sixty consecutive days after a hospital stay, the patient returns again to the hospital, Medicare coverage will begin anew—but the patient must have been out of the hospital at least sixty days in a row.

Part B is an optional supplement to Part A. If a patient chooses to pay the additional premium—$29.90 a month in 1991—Medicare pays some portion of a physician's fee and some of the cost of ambulances, transportation, braces, wheelchairs, artificial limbs, crutches, splints and casts, X-rays, laboratory tests, emergency room treatment in a hospital, outpatient hospital services, and some home health care.

The first $100, which is the deductible, is paid by the patient. Medicare pays 80 percent and the patient 20 percent of "reasonable charges" for services that are covered. Either the physician bills Medicare and the patient and gets part of his fee from each, or the patient pays the doctor and then has the burden of getting reimbursement from Medicare. It is better, and in the long run cheaper for the patient, when the physician bills Medicare. This is called "assignment."

Medicare pays for skilled nursing home care or rehabilitation for the same condition immediately following a hospitalization. "Skilled care" means the services of a registered or licensed practical nurse are necessary. Twenty days of full coverage are paid for. For the next eighty days, the patient must make a copayment of $78.50 a day. Another method of payment would be necessary beyond that period.

Medicare now provides benefits for home health care if the patient meets these eligibility requirements:

- The patient must be confined to the home.
- The patient's physician must determine that he needs home health care, such as skilled nursing care, physical therapy, or speech therapy.

243

- The physician must set up a care plan, or the home health agency providing services must participate in Medicare.

Medicare does not cover custodial nursing or homemaking services, nor do most "Medigap" policies from private insurance companies. (Some insurers, such as Prudential, do cover home care.) Medicare does not pay for the costs of meal preparation, general household services, shopping, or other home care services that assist people in meeting personal needs.

To avoid confusion about services covered by Medicare and to find out how to fill out a Medicare form, get a copy of "Your Medicare Handbook," a pamphlet available free at your local Social Security office; it describes the entire program in detail. A member of Medicare has a right to appeal and to protest a decision that he feels is unfair and to ask for a review through the Bureau of Hearings and Appeal. But be forewarned that dealing with the federal government is very time-consuming and may take several months. It may also be necessary to be represented by legal counsel when you appeal to a Medicare decision.

Medicare discriminates against people with diagnoses of Alzheimer's and similar diseases. If the confused person needs custodial care—that is, needs supervised help with meals and bathroom habits but does not need nursing care—Medicare will not cover these costs. The memory-impaired person may qualify only if he needs a nurse to review his medical status or to give an injection or change a catheter on a daily basis. These practices are unfair. (In the same vein, home health care aides caring for confused patients at home are covered by Medicare only if they are ordered by a physician.)

Medicare is of little help to nursing home residents since it only covers medical bills, and residents must become nearly destitute in order to qualify for Medicaid.

MEDICAID

Medicaid provides medical care for the indigent. It was added to the original Medicare bill at the last second. Medicaid is a state-run program even though its funds come from the U.S. government. Since each state designs its own program based on federal regulations, Medicaid varies greatly from state to state. You are eligible for Medicaid if you are (1) receiving public assistance (Home Relief), Aid for Dependent Children (AFDC), or Supplemental Security Income (SSI); (2) over age 65, blind or disabled, with low income; (3) over age 65, blind or disabled, with high medical expenses. Even if you have other health insurance coverage (such as Blue Cross/Blue Shield, HMO, or Medicare), Medicaid will pay whichever costs these policies do not cover.

If a person is eligible for SSI, he is also eligible for Medicaid, but he must fill out a separate form. Qualification for Medicaid is based on the amount of assets (property and savings) you have and the amount of income you receive, as well as on financial need. You must apply for Medicaid coverage for your memory-impaired relative through the Department of Welfare, the Department of Social Services, or the Health Department in your state. Always apply in writing to protect your rights.

Medicaid benefits entitle you to free health care from a physician, pharmacist, hospital, and other providers of health care who are specifically registered as providers of state Medicaid. Sometimes it is difficult to find health-care providers who accept Medicaid. You must determine in advance if the providers will accept Medicaid. If they do, present your monthly Medicaid card, which has a number. The physician will send a bill to Medicaid and receive reimbursement from the state.

Laboratory tests, X-rays, drugs, eyeglasses and eye examinations, dental services, prosthetic devices and surgical supplies, transportation and medical care, home care, and the services of doctors, clinics, hospitals, and nursing homes are all covered by Medicaid.

Documents to bring with you to determine eligibility for Medicaid include: written or printed proof of (a) your identity, (b) residence, (c) citizenship (or status as an alien), (d) income, (e) employment, (f) resources, (g) how you managed to care for the patient in the past.

Monthly *countable income* determines eligibility for Medicaid and is determined by filling out a budget sheet on which you may deduce expenses from gross income. *Earned income* is income the applicant works for. *Unearned income* is all other income, including savings and checking accounts, stocks, and bonds, and the cash value of life insurance policies.

Medicaid does not count some types of resources, including: (1) a home that is owned by you or your spouse as long as you live there, (2) income-producing real estate, (3) clothing and personal effects, (4) household furniture and appliances, (5) automobiles, (6) tools and equipment for employment purposes.

Some states, such as New York, have a *spend-down* program that can help a person reduce his resources and thus become eligible for Medicaid. For example, buying a new television set to replace one that doesn't work well will reduce the $2,900 of savings Mr. Carson has in his savings account by $450, leaving a total of $2,450, which is below the New York State eligibility level of $2,850 or less for an individual and $4,400 for a couple.

Many people enter a nursing home as private patients until their assets are reduced to the Medicaid eligibility level. They become eligible for Medicaid through this surplus-income or spend-down program, since their excess income is being spent on monthly medical care (nursing home costs).

> MR. DOBSON: "All I have is a house—worth maybe sixty-five thousand dollars—and my savings, which is about twenty thousand dollars. If my wife goes to the nursing home, all of our savings will be gone. The point is, we worked all our lives to have a little something, and it will be gone like that. Then how will I manage? I need something to live on, too."

Many spouses and children see the law mandating that married people bear permanent financial responsibility for each other's care as being unfair. It requires that couples use all the financial resources at their disposal (including what may have been intended for a comfortable old age or as an inheritance for the children) for medical expenses. Such a law springs from America's free enterprise medical system. In societies where health insurance is less costly, as in England and the Scandinavian countries, the elderly and infirm are better cared for without having to divest themselves of their life savings. However, taxes are very high in these countries to support their system of socialized medicine.

American health care is the best in the world, but the costs to maintain such quality are staggering. It is estimated that it costs the American public billions of dollars a year to institutionalize and care for the approximately 3.4 million victims of Alzheimer's disease and other forms of organic memory impairment. Usually it is the middle classes that are the hardest hit. The wealthy can afford to pay; the indigent are entitled to receive help.

Those people surviving primarily on Social Security but who have some assets should be aware of "deeming," a legal procedure that went into effect in some states in January 1977. Under this regulation the income and assets of the spouse who is not in an institution will be considered separately from those of the institutionalized spouse after one to six months of physical separation. Since 1989 states must allow sufficient income for the spouse who is not afflicted. The allowable household income for two people will be 150 percent of the federal poverty level as of July 1992. When the spouse living in the community refuses to pay, then the state must provide Medicaid to the spouse who is in the nursing home. Cases that have been taken by attorneys as far as the family courts have usually been won. Thus, those spouses who live predominantly on Social Security do not have to contribute to the cost of institutional care.

The middle classes must practically become impoverished before they can qualify for government assistance programs. Some are forced into deceiving the government in order to avoid financial bankruptcy. Transferring assets of the impaired person and spouse to children, other relatives, or friends in order to make the patient eligible for Medicaid is a frequently advised tactic. However, it may result in temporary ineligibility for public medical assistance. For example, a law that has taken effect in the state of New York states that as of April 10, 1982, Medicaid may be denied an applicant for two years if he transfers assets of $12,000 or less, and then be denied for an additional month for each $2,000 transferred in excess of $12,000, unless the applicant incurs medical expenses equal to the amount transferred. This is complicated and warrants the attention of an attorney knowledgeable about successful financial planning.

There are ways of counteracting the effect of such a law: setting up a trust fund, buying tax-free bonds, or, according to the Economic Recovery Tax Act of 1981, giving gifts of $10,000 per person per year to children or grandchildren, or an unlimited amount to a spouse.

COMBINING MEDICARE AND MEDICAID

If you have both state and federal coverage (Medicaid and Medicare), Medicaid will pay your annual $100 deductible and your 20 percent coinsurance fee under certain circumstances. If your doctor accepts *both* Medicaid and Medicare assignments, he or she agrees to accept 80 percent of what Medicare approves. You would usually have to pay the other 20 percent, plus your annual $100 deductible. Medicaid will pay it for you, however. (If your doctor does not want to participate in the Medicaid program, you will have to pay the extra expense yourself.) Thus, your best bet is to go to a doctor who accepts both. To find out which doctors accept Medicare assignments, check with your local Social Security (federal) or Medicaid (state) office. Doctors choose to accept Medicare assignments on a case-by-case basis.

Family Financial Considerations

To protect a family's funds from being totally dissipated in the care of a chronically ill patient, parents are sometimes advised to place their entire estate in trust, with one of their children named as conservator and themselves as beneficiaries. This is a perfectly legal and often a logical solution, but it may be a difficult one for parents to accept and to accomplish. Most of us find it uncomfortable to consider the possibility of our own incapacity or death and therefore tend to avoid making plans that acknowledge such a possibility. When children attempt to assume control of their parents' financial affairs, the parents sometimes feel threatened.

MRS. McHUGH: "I worked for my husband in his real estate business for many years. I did the bookkeeping, but he signed the checks. He started questioning every check I gave him to sign, because he would forget which bills had been paid, and his signature became almost illegible.

"When I saw this happening, I spoke to my son George. He suggested to my husband that we set up a trust fund for ourselves and let George manage it for us. My husband would have no part of it. He accused George of trying to grab the money for himself. 'Don't be so greedy,' he said. 'You'll get it all after I'm dead—that's soon enough!' Of course, by the time he died, the nursing home had taken nearly every penny. There's almost nothing for me to live on, and George won't get anything when I die."

Usually, when there is a trusting relationship between parents and children, parents are more willing to set up a fund similar to that proposed by George McHugh. However, some elderly parents do fear that once the children become the owners of the trust fund they will steal the money or spend it unwisely. Many elderly people are loath to rely on their children, especially when they are aware of some of the weaknesses in their children's character, or of rivalry among siblings.

Brothers and sisters may, in fact, vie with one another for an anticipated inheritance. As a strategy in such a competition, one of the children may take on the responsibility of major caregiver to an ailing parent. However, the parents' estate, whatever its size, is probably not actually the desired goal. The proportion of an inheritance symbolizes for a child the esteem in which his parents hold him and the value that they place on him. Therefore, the struggle among siblings is generally a struggle for power.

If you are a parent seeking to conserve your assets, both for your own support and for the benefit of your children, you must know the character of and trust the person who is appointed guardian of your funds. Even before you choose someone for this position, you should consult an attorney, a tax advisor, and a gerontologist who can advise you wisely before you make decisions about how to divest yourself of your funds.

Legal Matters

Competent legal advice is essential to prevent Alzheimer's patients and their families from facing economic depletion and the indignities of the erosion of individual rights. Estate planning can help ensure that institutionalization can be financed by Medicaid without making the spouse destitute. Medical care decisions, including the question of life-sustaining equipment, require that another person have legal authority to make such decisions.

Ethical issues concerning the legal capacity of an Alzheimer's patient, including his ability to make judgments and execute documents, often present legal problems. There may be disagreement among family members, or between a physician and family members.

Therefore, it is crucial to obtain competent legal advice whenever a person is diagnosed as having a form of dementia, including Alzheimer's disease. Some of the factors to consider include:

POWER OF ATTORNEY

Power of attorney is created when an adult (the client) signs a document that names another person as "attorney in fact." On behalf of his client, the attorney can act and sign documents, even after the client has been declared mentally incompetent. This transfer of power remains valid until the client's death.

LIVING OR INTER VIVOS TRUST

A living trust designates a member of the family to manage the patient's affairs when the patient and/or his spouse can no longer do so. It also protects privacy by allowing the terms of the will to remain private. A living trust includes a plan to distribute the Alzheimer's patient's assets after death; it also avoids the need for probate of a will or a conservatorship.

250

CONSERVATORSHIP OR GUARDIANSHIP

A conservatorship requires the court to oversee the patient's affairs in a protective way when there is no friend or relative to assume management. It also protects the impaired person from a self-interested or dishonest family member. A patient may petition for the court for a conservatorship by signing a document that appoints a person of his choice as a conservator for the future.

Relocating the Impaired Person

Once the decision is made to place your relative in a nursing home (or in any other sheltered setting where he will no longer be completely independent) and the financial arrangements have been concluded, the process of relocating must be accomplished with as little stress and confusion as possible.

For those of us whose memories are intact, a move or a change involves feelings of excitement and anticipation along with a sense of loss. When we have recently moved, we long temporarily for those places and friends we have left behind. For the impaired person, who may rely completely on the predictability of familiar surroundings and daily events to make sense of the world, the feeling of loss is magnified and the prospect of a new situation is frightening.

MR. PORTER: "I'm retired, and I'm comfortably well off. People ask me all the time why I don't sell my place here in Oak Park and move to someplace warm. My sister loves to be outdoors whenever it's warm enough, and she could do with a warm climate all year long. But, as I tell my friends, I would never, never move her into a new surrounding. She couldn't function as she does now. Here, she knows everyone in the neighborhood, and they know her. They know she has a problem, so they watch out for her and don't let her wander off too far or get lost. Every time she goes out she says hello to everyone, and they wave back. I'm pretty sure it makes her feel comfortable and secure. I couldn't move her away from all that is familiar to her."

At the present time, Mr. Porter has the ability to care for his sister in her own setting. Even if the time comes when he can no longer manage her care at home, his sensitivity to her need for familiar faces and objects will help him transfer her to an institution with a minimum of strain on her.

Memory-impaired people need familiar items and unchanged routines even more than the rest of us do, because they have lost the ability to learn new information. It helps to take along to the nursing home the small objects that still have meaning for the new resident: favorite photographs, a desk set or paperweight, a familiar robe and slippers that can be put on without help, anything that will give a sense of belonging in the new room and help keep the new resident from feeling abandoned. In fact, the person who is moving to the nursing home should have some say, if possible, about the items that he holds most dear. Some care must be taken, of course, to make sure he doesn't choose more things than the home can possibly accept.

No matter how difficult it may be to admit it, try to tell your confused relative that he is going to move, where he is going to live, and why he must be in a different place. Make the explanation as simple and gentle as possible. Perhaps he will forget what you have said. Even if you feel uncomfortable telling him over and over again about the move, your reminders and reassurances can ease some of his apprehension.

Occasionally families are advised not to prepare their patients for a move to a nursing home for fear that the very act of telling the patient may upset or enrage him. However, those spouses, siblings, and children who have shared in deceiving a patient in order to transport him to the nursing home ("Come on, Daddy, we're taking you out to dinner!") have felt enormous guilt afterwards.

The Patient's Adjustment

Adjustment to a nursing home is a two-fold process, requiring different and individual accommodations from the patient and the family.

For the patient, adjustment to a nursing home means learning the routines, who the roommate is, where things are put, what time meals are served, where the bathroom is, who can help with clothing, medication, and so on. The confused person will learn the procedure through staff members assigned to help with orientation to the new surroundings.

Sometimes there are severe setbacks in the patient's physical and/or mental health shortly after the move to a nursing home. The elderly person, perceiving that the move is intended to be a permanent one, may experience a sense of separation and loss that can lead to depression. Separation from family and one's own home has stressful effects on people of all ages. For the elderly, the stressful effect of separation may involve a feeling of final rejection and abandonment by family members and by all of society. Feeling extremely vulnerable, the elderly person may also experience many unconscious fears such as the threat of exposure and the fear of acting out his sexual impulses in an inappropriate context. These fears are related to the anxiety about being in a new and unfamiliar environment where there are new faces to get used to, different hands that touch you, unfamiliar rules and regulations, and rooms that are to be shared with strangers.

Depression may occur as soon as the elderly person is institutionalized. Sometimes rapid physical and emotional decline is apparent. These reversals may be temporary, however, and can improve with time. Don't panic and regret your decision to use the option of a nursing home. It would be unwise to take the elderly person out immediately, or move him elsewhere prematurely.

Adjustment to the nursing home is a process that can take as much as a year, although it is ideally accomplished in about six months. Some residents resign themselves to their fate, others become happier and more active, and some people, sadly, do not adjust at all and continue to decline physically and mentally. In many cases, the confused resident's loss of memory gives protection against anxiety, fear of abandonment, and a sense of loss. Since he cannot miss what he doesn't remember, the loss of memory can be a blessing in disguise for the impaired person. In this case, the patient's adjustment to the nursing home is swift. It is the family members who may become depressed and sustain excessive guilt feelings and strong reactions of grief.

A three-sided partnership incorporating the staff, the family, and the resident can be important in achieving a better understanding of the patient and his needs. The staff can provide care on a twenty-four hour basis. The family's visit provides practical supervision of the staff. Like a good supervisor, praise the staff for their attention to your relative whenever you can. They will show their appreciation for you and your relative by continuing good care. You and the rest of the family can maintain an intimate affection for the resident; the resident, where possible, can take responsibility for his own life.

A painful time for family members is when the confused patient asks to go home with them. Although it is heartbreaking and guilt-provoking to the relative, nursing home staff members are familiar with this behavior and know how to handle it without causing friction. They distract the patient by getting him ready for dinner or bed or by talking with him. Often a good rapport develops between the nursing home resident and an aide. This relationship is important to the patient, since he probably sees more of the aide than he does of his relative.

The Caregiver's Adjustment

Giving affection to a close friend or relative in a nursing home, and understanding his needs, can help that person feel cared for and important to others. Frequent visits offer continuity to the relationship, but so can telephoning and sending cards, letters, photographs, and newspaper clippings. The amount of our involvement with a relative in a nursing home depends on the strength of the ties in the old relationship, your current availability, and the needs of the resident.

You may find that your parent or spouse in the nursing home withdraws from you a little and finds new relationships in the home. Try not to be jealous of these connections. Some people handle the pain of separation by emphasizing new acquaintances. Newfound friends also help distract the person from negative feelings or from formerly destructive relationships.

Visits motivated by pity or guilt will make you irritable and annoyed with yourself; the patient will sense your feelings, and both of you may regret that the visit ever took place.

Self-involved, demanding parents, spouses, or relatives remain true to form in a nursing home. Learning to say no to such a person, even at this late juncture in life, is extremely important for the person who has been intimidated. Try not to become involved in power plays between the demanding, controlling resident and the staff. Set limits on yourself so that your time, energies, and emotions do not become drained. Eventually, your relative will get the message that this behavior no longer works with you, at which point, one hopes, it will stop.

Families or relatives who are overly solicitous of the nursing home patient may be motivated by guilt, fear of loss of inheritance, or competition with siblings or other relatives. Incessant complaints to staff members and interference with staff procedure is undermining to the patient. In reality, oversolicitousness may be a disguise for demanding behavior. It can be infuriating to the staff and destructive to the relative.

Some family members may demonstrate guilt and grief by rejecting their relatives, either openly or in more subtle ways, by decreasing their visits or not visiting at all. The pain of seeing the decline of a once-powerful parent or spouse makes us aware of our own mortality. We must face our own aging and the possibility that this could happen to us. The thoughts of the inevitability of the death of a loved one and ultimately of our own death are sometimes too much to bear. These are very powerful feelings from which many of us prefer to hide; but confronting these feelings with a good friend, an experienced counsellor or psychotherapist, or a supportive group can be extremely helpful and can strengthen us immeasurably.

Interaction with the staff should be cordial and respectful. If you abide by the rules and respect the nursing home's work schedules, you will earn the gratitude of the staff members. They, too, need your thanks; words of praise and appreciation are rewards that truly endure. Telling a supervisor about the superior performance or sensitivity of a nurse or aide toward your relative is equally important. It can mean a commendation that will be taken into consideration when that person's professional advancement is considered.

Think it over carefully before offering monetary rewards or tips to nursing home personnel. It is better to express gratitude and appreciation verbally or in a letter to the board of trustees or administrator of the home. Thanking someone in person gives him recognition and lets him know that his services are valued, while tipping may be demeaning and infer that only by offering payment can you be assured that your relative will receive the care to which he is entitled.

Even in the best of circumstances, crises may arise that make you want to take your relative back to your home or transfer him to another institution. You will need time to find a new home and to make a smooth transition. In the interim, report all infractions of the nursing home code and all setbacks of the resident to the administration of the home.

Friends and Relatives of the Institutionalized Aged (FRIA), located in New York, is an example of a watchdog group that looks into patient abuse or nursing home care abuse. Such a group can exert pressure on the administration of a home to improve whatever condition exists that is to the detriment of the home's residents.

Advocates for the elderly and nursing home reform groups around the country, including the Ad Hoc Coalition for a Single Standard Nursing Home Code, have already won an important consumer victory. The Reagan administration abandoned its plans to repeal important federal regulations protecting the rights of nursing home residents. Among these protected rights is the requirement that residents be treated with dignity and respect.

The serious problems that sometimes occur in nursing homes can intensify feelings of guilt in a caregiver.

Mrs. Santino reluctantly put her husband into a nursing home only after he became very belligerent and violent at home. In the first six weeks after his admission, he seemed more placid and compliant with the staff. Even so, Mrs. Santino worried about him, but when she prolonged her visits through the dinner hour, the staff asked her to leave. She kept trying to force her husband to eat, and this disrupted the nursing home routine.

Mrs. Santino acceded to the staff's request. Shortly thereafter, she noticed that her husband looked very thin. She alerted the head nurse, who told her that although Mr. Santino would eat breakfast, he refused any food the rest of the day, and that he was being fed a liquid diet to make up for the food he missed. Mrs. Santino was perplexed—why wouldn't he eat? She inquired further and learned that an orderly to whom Mr. Santino was particularly responsive had been transferred to another shift. There seemed to Mrs. Santino to be a direct relationship between her husband's "hunger strike" and the loss of the orderly who was able to elicit a response from him.

Beside herself with grief, Mrs. Santino blamed herself for having put her husband in the nursing home where such things could happen. The nursing home would not force him to eat, as she would have at home. She cried and felt the gnawing pangs of guilt: "They're not trying to make him eat. He'll die of malnutrition! I feel like a murderer because I put him in the nursing home!"

When she expressed these feelings to her therapist, it was apparent that her panic was related to the enormous guilt she felt for relieving herself of the burden of caring for her husband.

Mrs. Santino became somewhat calmer when she understood that the nursing home would not allow her husband to die of malnutrition. Although it was unlikely that the orderly who could cajole Mr. Santino to eat would be reinstated to his old nursing station, the staff would supplement Mr. Santino's diet with extra calories and feed him liquids if he continued to refuse food. If extreme measures were necessary, the staff would nourish him by feeding him through a tube in his nose. Mrs. Santino wept bitterly at the prospect and berated herself for her heartlessness, until gradually she was able to see that there were no other possible alternatives: she could not manage her husband's care at home; the nursing home was doing the best that could be done. She would have to "live through" her grief, expressing it verbally and trying actively to mitigate it.

Mrs. Santino eased her guilt somewhat by spending many hours in the nursing home helping her husband and his fellow patients. When she travelled home in the evening, although fatigued and somewhat depressed, she was relieved that she could look forward to a chat with her neighbor, an uninterrupted dinner, and a peaceful night's sleep. Gradually, she settled into a routine of visiting her husband as part of her life, making time for him as well as for other things in her life.

257

The Step-by-Step Approach to Appropriate Patient Care in Nursing Homes

Since the Alzheimer's patient has a significant recent-memory failure, step-by-step teaching and repetition of such skills as bathing, dressing, and hair combing may ensure that these skills are not lost prematurely. If these skills are not used, they will surely be forgotten. Encouraging patients to do as many activities of daily living for themselves as possible helps the patient to maintain independence for as long as possible.

Prior to nursing home acceptance, a preadmission home visit is essential. At that time the patient's functional abilities can be ascertained. The assessment should be ongoing and repeated within a few days of nursing home admission. Within two to four months, the assessment can be repeated. This will help to determine when a chronic condition has become exacerbated into an acute episode.

It is important to individualize each Alzheimer's patient so that he is not expected to have skills that he is incapable of performing. Step-by-step directions by staff members who offer assistance to patients when they forget enable patients to continue self-care. (See Chapter 12 for more on this technique.)

Many nursing homes, but not all, have special Alzheimer's disease units. They must be spacious to allow the patient physical mobility. They should be on the ground level with easy access to an enclosed garden or outdoor area in which patients can walk but be protected in case they wander. Moving about freely and feeling the change of air as seasons change may improve the patient's ability to orient himself in time and place.

Predictability is a key to helping the patient remain oriented. Routine times for meals, going to bed, and getting up, as well as allowing attachments to the same personnel, provide consistency and stability and give structure to the Alzheimer's patient's turmoil. Habit then will supplant memory loss.

Orderliness, calmness, and safety precautions all contribute to beneficial patient-staff interaction. Telling the patient what to do in a simple, quiet tone, such as, "We are going to the lounge now," and "Now is the time to eat breakfast," will preclude outbursts or fearful responses in the patient. Life is lived in the existential moment for the Alzheimer's patient. It must also be so for the staff and the patient's visitors.

Other Alternatives to Your Home or a Nursing Home

In the early stages of Alzheimer's disease a patient and his family can benefit from such programs as a visiting nurse service and Meals on Wheels. There are other services for patients who need more attention.

ADULT DAY CARE CENTERS

Day care for a few hours a day may be a suitable alternative for your relative and may also provide enough respite for you to enable you to continue to care for him at home. Sometimes the staff of a day hospital or day care center consists of physicians, nurses, and physical therapists. Lunch, opportunity for socializing with other patients, and medical care (when necessary) are all provided. Patients with Alzheimer's disease are not segregated but integrated into the program.

Day care is a viable alternative to institutionalizing an Alzheimer's victim. It affords family caregivers opportunities for rest or continuing to work during the day. Also, the flexibility of day care in terms of hours and days per week can suit the needs of the caregivers. Family caregivers often volunteer at day care centers and learn skills that can be used with the Alzheimer's patient at home.

Social stimulation and change of atmosphere are two important benefits to the Alzheimer's patient. Social interaction with other people offers opportunities for learning that meets the individual's capacities and existing skills. Day care can become a familiar and pleasant routine that uplifts the mood of the Alzheimer's patient and carries over to the home.

The caregiver has the opportunity to be with the Alzheimer's patient as he chooses, thereby satisfying his needs to be with the patient without

259

the burden of twenty-four hour care. When full-time home care is too burdensome, day care can provide a step before institutionalization that is less emotionally painful for the caregiver. Day care provides relief and is the bridge between these two types of care.

Although day hospitals and day care centers vary, they usually include a program of reality orientation in which patients are encouraged to know the day, date, month, year, their own names, and so forth. There are helpful, stimulating discussions about memory impairment, and reminiscing over old photographs is invited. Music and dancing are used to evoke memories and emotions. During the course of the day there are opportunities to play memory games, to play bingo using pictures, and to discuss stories about families. Supervised exercises help to release energy and control the patients' restlessness, and communicating with other patients is encouraged. The emphasis is always on what the patient is able to do. The team of specialists provides guidance, structure, and support for confused and disoriented elderly participants. Equally important, the concerned family can supplement the day care center's efforts by continuing to use reality orientation at home and remaining supportive to the patient. Fees for such services are often on a sliding scale and may range from $15 to $60 per day, plus $10 per day for transportation. Medicaid rarely covers the cost of day care.

FOSTER CARE

There are other living situations that may be viable and more appealing than a nursing home. For the most part, they are suitable only for the mildly impaired person. They also tend either to be expensive or to be in such demand that waiting lists are very long. The least expensive of these situations is foster care, which is generally paid for by the state.

Patients with moderate memory lapses and mild disorientation are usually more effectively treated at home, or in a foster home or home for the aged. Elderly people may, like some children, be placed in foster homes and given a room, meals, transportation to medical facilities, and supervision. Foster families are paid by the state to care for the elderly, who are treated as members of their foster families. Of course, the genuineness of the foster family's attitude toward the older person helps to determine the adequacy of this alternative living arrangement.

BOARD AND CARE HOMES

Still relatively inexpensive, but offering a higher level of skilled nursing care, are halfway houses or homes for the elderly run by state hospitals, churches, or synagogues.

Sheltered housing, which may or may not have subsidized rents for the elderly, depending on how it was funded, offers conveniences such as wheelchair ramps, grab bars, and other safety features for physically disabled older people. Although a nurse and a social worker are usually on staff, such living situations provide no special help for the memory-impaired.

LIFE-CARE COMMUNITIES

For those who have sufficient capital, the choice of living situation is wider. Life-care institutions are residential settings that require both an entrance fee and either monthly maintenance charges or a fee for service, which the facility invests and from which it makes a profit. In return for this investment, care is provided for the remaining life span of the individual. As he becomes increasingly disabled, he is moved to more protective and skilled nursing care. Other possible choices for the relatively wealthy, self-sufficient elderly include a senior citizens' hotel or "retirement community."

STATE HOSPITALS

A patient with Alzheimer's disease may have to be placed in the geriatric unit of a state mental hospital if his condition is so extreme that nursing homes refuse to admit him. Nursing homes have a limited ability to control constant wandering, so they may refuse to take a patient who is perpetually trying to leave, to force his way outside, or to struggle against those who attempt to keep him in the room. Nursing homes are also unprepared for exceptionally violent patients. A few Alzheimer's victims are seized with daily uncontrollable violent outbursts in which they may kick, punch, bite, or otherwise assault anyone in range, including the caregiver, unless physically restrained. Such patients are too disruptive both for home care and for most nursing homes. A state institution is then the most appropriate choice. The state mental hospital will usually have a staff skilled in geriatric medicine and, ideally, some skilled nursing care. Placing a relative in a state hospital does not eliminate the family's financial responsibility for the care of the patient, although the actual cost for care is much less than it is at either a nonprofit or a proprietary home. A spouse will be required to pay for care, and his assets will be considered in the same way that they would have been if the impaired spouse were in a nursing home.

The federal government has mandated that state hospitals reduce their geriatric patient load; thus, the hospital in your state may not wish to accept a new patient, especially with Alzheimer's disease. While state hospitals generally provide a poorer quality of care, some do have better organized facilities and staff, and there are some programs for the memory-impaired patient. You will need the signatures of a psychiatrist and a physician to have your relative admitted to a state mental hospital; you may need the assistance of a politician to get a bed for your relative.

If your relative does enter a state hospital, continue to show loving family concern and involvement by visiting frequently, just as you would if he were in a nursing home.

HOSPICES

Hospices are intended for people who doctors say have a limited amount of time to live, such as six months or less. At a hospice everything is aimed at making those last months more comfortable. Patients are treated with enormous kindness. Medical care focuses on relieving their pain and anxiety. Family members are offered counseling. In contrast to those hospitals with a mission of prolonging life no matter how empty it may become, hospices allow a patient to die naturally and peacefully.

Some aspects of hospice care are also available at home through visiting nurses and other services; this arrangement allows a patient to spend his last months in a familiar and loving place, surrounded by loved ones.

Visiting

When you visit your relative or spouse in a nursing home, act as interested in the patient and the environment as you would if you were visiting him in his own home. Sometimes all that is required of you is to ask a question, then listen attentively to the answer. Let your relative know in this way that his personality and opinions are still important to you.

There may be times when you may feel unrewarded by your visit.

Ms. Fuchs: "I had a very dear friend who was finally forced to put her mother in a nursing home. My friend would visit her mother every other day. She had a sister and a brother, both of whom worked full-time and spent evenings at home with their families, so my friend was the only one who visited regularly. And her mother could never remember if she was there. Her mother would say, 'You never visit! What a rotten daughter you are!' and she would answer quietly, 'But mother, I was just here yesterday.' It made no difference to her mother, but my friend went anyway."

It may not seem to make any difference to the patient, but it probably does. Most important, it makes a difference to the visitor, who would feel very guilty if she didn't see her mother often.

When you visit, you may be able to help your relative with personal care or exercise. Reminiscing about past events and experiences may be an excellent way to share the time. Enrich your visits by sharing such simple pleasures as a meal or listening to music. If you enjoy walking together, visit a nearby store. Feed the birds in the garden; look at and smell the flowers.

In your visits, be verbally affectionate and give tender touches and embraces. If your young or teenage child wishes to visit, prepare him in advance for some of the depressing sights he may encounter. If he is prepared, the visit will give the child an opportunity to see life in another dimension. And for the impaired relative, having a young visitor will most likely afford delight and a sense of continuity with life outside the nursing home.

Caring for and sharing ourselves with those who are helpless is an opportunity for us to enlarge the emotional and spiritual nature of our own humanity. Those who are unable to face up to misfortune are perhaps unluckier; they must grieve in their own way.

CHAPTER 14

Death and Bereavement

Law, custom, and necessity require us to make plans for our own death. We make wills to distribute our possessions, to ensure a certain amount of financial security for our relatives when possible, and to make our posthumous wishes known. If we choose to donate our organs for scientific research, we must make a clear and legal declaration of our intent. When a confused, memory-impaired relative can no longer make these decisions for himself, we must act on his behalf.

However, you must be legally empowered to do so. While he is still capable of executing a legal document, obtain a power of attorney. This will be necessary before you can take over his bank accounts or sign his legal papers. Some patients give power of attorney willingly. Those who are more confused, suspicious, or paranoid resist but often can be persuaded by the family lawyer, an insurance agent, a business partner, or other associates whom the impaired person respects and trusts.

The power of attorney also helps you gain access to your patient's assets (such as safety deposit boxes and individual savings accounts). In addition it gives you the authority to determine the disposition of your patient's body after his death.

Putting a Patient's Affairs in Order

Whether you need the loved one's assets in order to provide for his care or to make an assessment of his estate after his death, you may be faced with the problem of searching for lost, mislaid, or hidden items of which you are ignorant or about which the confused person has forgotten. Logical places, like desk drawers and offices, may turn out to be the wrong places to look. You may have to comb the impaired person's apartment or house and look in unlikely places to find a will, bank books, stock certificates, bonds, insurance policies, keys, address books, or receipts. A confused person may put these valuable items anywhere. Keep looking, especially if you suspect that not all the important papers have been recovered.

When people become forgetful, their resources and debts are forgotten. While debts will eventually surface, assets do not turn up so easily.

Ida Cohen told us that she searched every nook and cranny in the kitchen, bedroom, and bathroom for information on her husband's bank accounts. She even tried the piano bench and the radiators, to no avail. But one day while getting some ice from the freezer, she came across small rolled-up pieces of paper with numbers on them. She figured out that her husband had written the numbers of his bank accounts on these papers, rolled them up, and put them in the freezer for "safety." These numbers could have remained in the deep freeze, with Ida none the wiser. Indeed, her husband's considerable assets were staring her in the face each time she opened her freezer door. These and similar stories show that the suspiciousness of Alzheimer's patients contributes to their bizarre behavior.

If your relative has been in the service, contact the military to see what benefits a veteran's dependents may be eligible for. Check for retirement and disability benefits via cancelled checks. Apply for Social Security benefits, union benefits, and pensions from the state or federal government.

In addition, look for insurance policies that may pay lump-sum benefits. Premium notices should give the name of the company your relative was insured with. Mutual funds, certificates of deposit, or stock certifi-

266

cates may be found through records of purchase or sale or the name of the broker. Look for correspondence in these matters.

Business, rental, or leased property may be traced through tax forms, keys, or notices about tax assessments. Insurance agents can help. Also, public records reveal real estate property ownership.

Assets may include safety deposit boxes, so look for a key or a bank receipt. You need a court order to open someone else's property. Gold, jewelry, cash, antique furniture, cars, or gems may also be hidden in wall or floor safes or in storage places. Look for a key, or check the least likely places in the home of the deceased.

The deceased may also have had foreign bank accounts, a trust fund or inheritance, or a personal loan due him that is still outstanding. Evidence of these can be found in bank statements, divorce agreements, interest statements, and correspondence. The person may have also purchased a cemetery plot. Look for a receipt of payment.

A will should list all of a person's assets. Sometimes wills are filed with an attorney or placed in a safety deposit box.

Making plans for yourself or your Alzheimer's patient *before* you reach the point of no return mentally will save your relatives the time, burden, and emotional trauma of having to search for documents, keys, and so on. We often make such plans before an airplane or car journey. Preparing for death should be part of life. One can arrange for a funeral or cremation and for disbursement of one's assets and precious possessions. Taking these steps can bring us spiritual peace and comfort, knowing that we are in control of our destiny for as long as humanly possible. It is the poetry of death that, as Dylan Thomas wrote, we may "rail against the dying of the light," but we accept death when it comes. Then the spirit and the soul can be at peace.

Anticipatory Grief

Grief may be prolonged and extended over a period of time. Where there has been a long illness, such as Alzheimer's disease or a similar condition, the spouse or children may mourn in advance. This anticipatory grief is a protective device that prepares the caregiver for his loss.

The opportunity to prepare in anticipation of bereavement may have a profoundly helpful effect upon the caregiver's subsequent reaction to the death of a loved one. However, even though we know a relative is dying, we sometimes suppress our anticipatory grief for fear of upsetting the dying person. The husband who shares his thoughts and plans about his dying wife, and begins to anticipate what life will be like without her, is in a better position to cope with bereavement than the one who pretends the spouse is going to continue living.

Sadness is a component of anticipatory grieving. Even if you mourn for a substantial period of time while your relative still lives, such grieving may never be completed because of unpredictable feelings that may arise.

When there has been a great deal of anticipatory grieving and advance mourning, however, the survivors may feel relieved, and thus no longer feel the need to mourn, when the actual death occurs. In such a situation, the period of mourning and readjustment may be shorter and less painful than for families who are unable to plan for the death of a loved one.

Grieving

The relationship between Alzheimer's disease and other physical illnesses is not fully understood. However, patients with Alzheimer's disease seem to be more susceptible than the rest of the elderly population to viruses, influenza, and pneumonia. These communicable diseases affect the Alzheimer's patient more severely than they do people who are not memory-impaired. Due to his apparent vulnerability, the Alzheimer's victim's life expectancy is reduced by one-third, in spite of his frequently youthful appearance and otherwise good physical health.

Despite the best care that can be given, patients die of Alzheimer's disease. This event causes a great emptiness in the life of the caregiver. Hours that had been filled with countless chores and duties now become vacant. Silence and stillness replace your busyness. When the anticipated death of your impaired relative becomes a reality, you may still find yourself deeply grieved even though you may already have been grieving during his lifetime. Grief is part of the normal mourning process; it is a basic human experience.

The first stage of grieving may be shock that the person has died. The bereaved relative may deny the death or event. This can lead to an agitated state of depression. Acute mourning may follow, an intense period in which the bereaved withdraws socially and may identify with the deceased person. The bereaved person may show an abnormal anxiety over his health and develop imaginary illnesses (hypochondriacal behavior), which can be accompanied by severe melancholic behavior. The third stage may be a resolution. Bereaved men and women who do not complete the last stage of mourning often become chronic mourners. They do not permit themselves pleasure or any cessation of the mourning process.

The task of mourning is gradually to surrender the psychological attachment to a deceased loved one. During the period of bereavement, the bonds of affection to the deceased are gradually loosened. Intense grief reactions generally last between three and twelve weeks, and the mourning process usually continues between one and two years. When the mourning period is over, we usually assume that the bereaved has "worked through" the loss and freed himself from the intense attachment to the unavailable person. As a result of the loss, the bereaved person may experience significant emotional and behavioral changes.

Being in a state of bereavement—that is, mourning, instead of avoiding the suffering—offers a person the opportunity to become psychologically ready, or at liberty, to try a fresh, new, and meaningful relationship. After a loss, the crucial factors in recovery from the loss include good health, a capacity for intelligent decision-making, and freedom from emotional disorders. Unfortunately, many people allow themselves to decline following the loss of a loved one. The decline may include a breakdown in physical health, losses of money or possessions, isolated social status, and changes in appearance. (Some people claim that their hair has actually turned gray overnight.)

Elderly men and women who become widowed often suffer various forms of grief. The grief may be inhibited or disguised; it is then expressed in physical symptoms, by isolating themselves from others, or by over-identifying with the lost loved one. In certain cases, bereaved people may be openly hostile toward another living person. Some widowed people may develop the irrational belief that their spouses died on purpose, thus rejecting their love. This belief, although unreasonable, can lead to guilty feelings, apathy, irritability, hostility, or hyperactivity. The survivors may also develop psychosomatic complaints (physical ailments) or imitations of the physical symptoms that caused the death of the spouse. Often the widowed are total unaware of any connection between their physical symptoms and their grief.

The purpose of grief and mourning is to accept the reality of the loss and begin to find new ways of filling up the emptiness caused by the loss. Widows and widowers are greatly relieved when they are told that once they resolve their grief, the symptoms of illness will gradually disappear.

Some people experience morbid grief reactions when they delay mourning for months or years. The person who is unable to cry at the funeral or thereafter may be experiencing such a delay in grieving. This is usually the result of either conscious or unconscious feelings of antagonism toward the dead person. Ambivalence (having conflicting positive and negative feelings at the same time) toward a deceased loved one may also cause delays in grieving. Negative and angry feelings toward the deceased person during his lifetime or excessive guilt about the loss of love for the dead person may prevent a resolution of grieving.

As older people begin to review their lives and the things they have or haven't done, sometimes they begin to blame themselves a great deal. Expiation and atonement must begin at once, because time is running out. Fences must be mended—that is, old grudges put aside and reparations made for past unkindness. The hope for forgiveness from relatives and friends stems from the need to resolve guilt. It is an essential aspect of finally accepting our lives as worthwhile.

Attempts at making reparations to another person can be made if the person is alive, willing, and available to receive them. If not, then only by talking about guilt and other painful feelings will mourners be able to complete their mourning and atonement. Then they may go on about the business of living, which includes identifying with a new style of life, discovering new people, and having pleasurable experiences.

Emotional isolation, or locking oneself up inside, makes us prisoners of our own fears and anxieties. It does not allow us to obtain the warmth and comfort that is available from others. Isolating oneself may be a way of being faithful to the old love tie. Many divorced people, as well as the widowed, handle their grief in this way. Unfortunately, they are preventing themselves from making new and satisfying bonds that can be established over time.

Survivor Guilt

If your patient dies, only the physical relationship ends. It does not end the memory of the relationship, nor the feelings that the relationship evoked. These live on in the survivor's mind as he struggles toward some understanding of the often unanswerable and toward resolutions that may never be found. Why did I survive? Why am I not afflicted with the same illness? Why me? Doubts, blame, and finally, some pervasive feelings of guilt ensue over an unrepayable debt to the deceased.

"Survivor guilt" is a term that is usually reserved for people who have outlived their peers or spouses. It is also associated with those who have witnessed the mass killing of family members and friends, as in the Holocaust, Hiroshima, or Vietnam. The survivor is often left with an irrational but persistent sense of guilt about having survived.

Professional researchers who have studied survivor guilt suggest that the guilt referred to is really the memory of our own helplessness in the face of death. It may also be some recognition that society does not value the elderly. If we even inadvertently believe in the American cultural value system that extols youth and in which there is little evidence of reverence for the lives of the aged, then we may all share some survivor guilt.

Family members of chronically ill patients often bear the pain of chronic sorrow and guilt over the handicaps of their relatives. Intense grief feelings are reawakened and continually experienced as patients begin to deteriorate. Such feelings are normal reactions to abnormal situations. As the patient declines, the family's need for emotional support and information about managing the patient becomes increasingly important. Energetic network support systems are vitally important to the family caregiver to help alleviate some of the difficulties that he or she may encounter at these times.

Autopsy

Planning what to do after the death of a loved one may seem very callous while the person still lives. However, just as we plan how to distribute our wealth after our demise, it is important to plan for the disposal of the body and any subsequent procedures to be carried out. In a situation where a relative cannot plan for himself, the caregiver takes on the major responsibility.

To keep things from going awry, it is important to check state laws in advance. Have a notarized letter from your patient or from his next of kin (or whoever has his power of attorney) if it is your desire that his brain be donated for research purposes. This letter must be deposited with the medical director's office of the hospital where the autopsy will be performed. Studying the brain tissue of a suspected Alzheimer's patient is the only way to make a definitive diagnosis of Alzheimer's or other related diseases. An autopsy can also provide useful information that benefits science and furthers our knowledge of memory impairment. However, if your religious beliefs or those of the patient preclude such a procedure, decline the request.

For the surviving spouse, sibling, or child, the end of mourning brings the promise of new experiences and new relationships that can offer different, but very satisfying, life arrangements, and an opportunity to shift focus from the burden of love to its pleasures and joy.

Critical Issues for Professionals
with Aging Patients

The process of growing older brings with it declines in many of our prized capabilities. In addition to these losses, we begin to reexamine relationships as we get older. Ideally, this leads to a realistic acceptance of ourselves and, in turn, acceptance of others.

Professionals can also be adult children of aging parents or other relatives. Although we are adults, we are also children who may be struggling with the unique conflict of accepting the decline of aging parents. This often brings up the dilemma of confronting unresolved childhood issues. Did we feel loved enough? Accepted? Are we angry at our parents for hurting us, not having confidence in us, making inordinate demands on us, liking our siblings better, not showing affection? Can we tell our parents how we feel about them? Do we still need them to be supportive of us, tell us what to do, help us to make difficult decisions? Are we, the adult children, now put in the position of having to make decisions for our parents? Care for them? Are the parent and child roles now reversed? Must you protect your fragile parent whom you once honored and revered? Do you have conflicting loyalties to your own ambitions or your spouse or children and to your parents? Are you confused with demands for efficient management of your time and energy? Thus, sandwiched between such dilemmas, how can you improve your relationships within your own and your extended families?

Now revert back to your professional role as the office nurse, the physician, the gerontologist. You must find a way to accept the dependent position of your patients while understanding their desire and attempts to maintain their independence. With this group of patients and their families, you may find yourself in the role of an educator about the aging process. In your own life you must confront the fact that separation from loved ones is a developmental task that confronts us throughout life but particularly toward the end of an older adult's life. We must, through intellectual understanding and emotional acceptance, resolve our attitudes and feelings about separation and death.

273

PART THREE

Take Care
of Yourself

"Physician, heal thyself!"
—Luke 4:23

CHAPTER 15

Safeguard Your Health

Ms. SARAH DREYSON: "My great uncle had what they used to call hardening of the arteries, and we in the family always say that his illness killed his second wife. Aunt Celia became exhausted from going out in the middle of the night to fetch him home when he went wandering around without his clothes on. She felt so ashamed of his behavior, and got so upset whenever she had to go collect him at the police station, that she finally had a heart attack."

Celia Dreyson's family, like some others, blames the patient for the health problems of the caregiver. Caring for a person with Alzheimer's disease certainly puts an extraordinary stress on all one's physical and mental resources. It is for this very reason that the most loving care of your memory-impaired relative must include loving care for yourself. There are probably many ways that Aunt Celia could have lightened her burden. She could have reduced the effects of her own exhaustion and stress by looking after her physical health—by eating a well-balanced diet, getting regular medical attention, and understanding and learning to cope with the many upsetting and complex feelings that caregivers experience.

A Nutritious Diet

When you eat meals with a memory-impaired person, it's sometimes difficult to remember that, just as your relative needs a well-balanced, nourishing diet, you too must eat regularly and healthfully. By the time you have prepared food that your confused relative is willing to eat, helped him cut his meat or use his spoon, persuaded him to swallow properly and not to spit out the food, then cleaned up after his meal—and while cleaning up answered his repeated question "When do we eat?" it's not surprising if the last thing you want to think about is meal planning and food for yourself. There is a great temptation to settle for a TV dinner, to grab a snack of candy or crackers, or to skip eating altogether.

However, if you succumb too often to the impulse to skimp on your own nutrition, not only will you be endangering you own health, you will also be doing a great disservice to your impaired relative who depends on you for sustenance. To continue giving your relative good care, you need to nourish yourself properly.

In Chapter 10, when we talked about eating problems that your impaired relative may face, we mentioned some of the conditions that can result from nutritional deficiencies, such as chronic constipation, brittle bones, diabetes, heart disease, stroke, and mental confusion. If you're not eating properly, you are every bit as susceptible to these conditions as the person for whom you are caring. While good nutrition is not a way to avoid aging or death, which is inevitable for all of us, it may help us to avoid some of those ailments that are commonly associated with old age. It can be an important factor in whether we remain lively, well, active, and productive.

At the same time, we understand that it may not be a simple matter to serve yourself regular meals that fulfill the requirements of a proper diet. This is especially true if you are older yourself, living on retirement income or Social Security, weakened by illness, or limited by physical disabilities. It's also difficult to fix a meal when you're depressed, or when you must sit down to eat it in loneliness because your confused relative can't eat with you or doesn't talk to you anymore.

If, for whatever reason, you are not eating nourishing meals, you are not alone. Millions of elderly people throughout America are poorly nourished, according to Dr. Robert N. Butler, former director of the National Institute of Aging: "Federal food consumption studies suggest that the diets of the elderly are substandard, both in quality and in quantity."

Some of the reasons are economic. Inflation and the cost of living hit the elderly harder than any other age group. There are millions of elderly people who live below the poverty level. Social Security was never intended to provide the whole of a person's retirement income, although in too many cases it does so today.

Despite government programs, malnutrition is said to be implicated in 83 percent of all deaths of people over the age of 65. With inflation, a fixed income buys less; what food one can afford may have more fillers and less nutrients. When you shop for one or two people, you must generally buy smaller quantities, which cost more per serving; on the other hand, buying a giant economy size and having to discard half the package because it has spoiled is even less thrifty.

Other reasons for poor nutrition are health-related. If you have trouble chewing, for instance, or wear ill-fitting dentures, you may be tempted to rely on processed foods that are easy to chew but high in calories and low in proper nutrients. You may also eat less of everything than you should, because food is too difficult to chew. People with chronic illnesses whose concomitant effects include secondary digestive disturbances may restrict their diets and in the process deprive themselves of good food. Those who must follow a fat-free, sugar-free, or salt-free diet sometimes find it so difficult or boring that they inadvertently reduce their intake of other nutrients as well.

Food Preparation Services

Perhaps you can take advantage of the alternatives to solitary eating that are offered by a variety of nutrition programs found in most communities. Under the Older Americans Act, the federal government has funded nutrition sites and various Eating Together Congregate Meals and Home-Delivered Meals programs. One nutritious hot meal a day (mostly lunch, sometimes dinner) is provided at a nutrition center, sometimes a senior citizen center, which may be located in a local church, synagogue, or school. Often these centers offer, in addition to a hot meal, a variety of recreational projects. These can provide you with the opportunity to socialize during and after mealtimes in the company of others like yourself, usually at only a short distance from home. Where distances are great, transportation can often be provided.

Contact your local Office of Aging or Department of Social Services, Welfare, or Human Resources to find out more about these programs. Many such programs are free; some require that the participant pay for them on a sliding scale, or at a nominal charge. They are open to people over the age of 59 and their spouses, regardless of income level.

You may be able to take part in Meals on Wheels, a program for the elderly who are housebound. Once a day a hot meal is prepared and delivered to your home by a local volunteer through the auspices of a program or agency. Costs vary throughout the country: some communities may serve a hot meal five days a week for as little as $2.00 per week; others may charge $2.00 to $3.00 per meal.

Commercial (profit-making) home-delivery food services are available in some parts of the country, and some restaurants will prepare take-out meals. Unfortunately, these services are often prohibitive in cost for people with limited finances.

The importance to your health of having a hot meal delivered every day is apparent. In addition, you can enjoy the friendliness and companionship of the person who brings the food. This daily connection to the outside world can be very restorative, and as nourishing to your spirit as the meal is to your body.

Your neighbors, friends, and family members who live nearby are often more willing than you might think to help you to eat well, by making extra portions when they cook their own meals and bringing the food to you. This is a true act of kindness and a gift of love.

SOME BASIC PRINCIPLES

Although as we age we need fewer calories, we still need the same proportion of nutrients. Diet is a matter of individual nutritional needs and preferences; food intake may vary from day to day. However, to achieve a balanced diet we should count our calories, eat plenty of fibrous foods for roughage (whole grains, fruits, and vegetables are recommended), and ingest adequate amounts of foods rich in calcium (milk, yogurt, cottage cheese, spinach, collard greens, sardines, salmon, and molasses).

We should avoid junk foods, too much sugar, and excessive (or megadoses of) vitamins and minerals or other supplements. We should also be careful about the chronic use of any laxatives, diuretics, antibiotics, or anti-inflammatory drugs, all of which can lead to a depletion of essential minerals and vitamins in our bodies. Frequently there are natural substitutes available. Prunes and other dried fruits are known to have laxative properties. Warm milk can be an antidote to sleeplessness—the amino acid in it acts as a natural tranquilizer to the body.

A sufficiently balanced diet can be accomplished even when there is little variation in the menu. Nutrition experts now suggest that the simplest daily diet with adequate nutrients should be based on the Food Guide Pyramid that the U.S. Department of Agriculture released in April 1992:

- Six to eleven servings of bread, cereal, rice, and pasta
- Two to three servings of milk, yogurt, and cheese
- Two to three servings of meat, poultry, fish, eggs, dry beans, and nuts
- Three to five servings of vegetables
- Two to four servings of fruit
- Fats, oils, and sweets should be used sparingly

Rice should be combined with dry beans because each nutrient by itself is not a complete protein; together they constitute a complete protein.

To maintain your ideal weight, eat a variety of foods but avoid a lot of sodium (salt), saturated fat, cholesterol, and sugar. If you enjoy alcoholic beverages, drink moderately. Eat foods that have starch and fiber and foods with proteins and B vitamins—these are considered nourishers of the nervous system and the brain. Avoid TV dinners; they are usually high in salt, low in vitamins, and lack roughage. Prepackaged Weight-Watchers dinners have essential nutrients and are low in calories but may also exceed your food budget.

If you are worried about weighing too much and want a "painless" method to eat less and not feel hungry, you might be intrigued by these suggestions.

- Eat *breakfast* every morning to activate your metabolism at the beginning of each day.
- Choose more fruit, pasta, or vegetables when you eat. These are complex carbohydrates and tend to make you feel full.
- Drink twelve 8-ounce glasses of water per day. With 96 ounces of water in your stomach, it will stay fuller.
- Every three to four hours eat a small meal to speed up your metabolism and help you to stay full.
- Eat high water content foods that make you feel full.
- Use whole grains as a preferred source of starches, or complex carbohydrates.
- Fresh or dried foods are preferable to those foods with chemical preservatives such as sulphites.

The percentage of calories from protein can be 10 to 12 percent and from fat 20 to 25 percent but 60 to 70 percent should come from complex carbohydrates. The complex carbohydrates are whole-grain cereals, brown rice, millet, oats, barley, buckwheat, corn, rye, bulgar, whole-grain bread, kasha, popcorn, or starchy tubers such as yams.

If you are still uncertain about what to eat or how much to serve yourself (or your relative) because you have never before been responsible for making nutritious meals or supervising meal preparation, or if you don't have confidence in your ability to plan your own menu, consult a home economics teacher, a public health nurse, or a nutritionist or registered dietician (R.D.). Usually, an R.D. has completed a course of study in dietetics from an accredited college or university and has worked as a dietician in a school or hospital. A consulting dietician can provide either general nutrition advice or an easy-to-follow menu plan with a particular selection of foods suitable to your needs if you have a specific ailment such as obesity, diabetes, liver disease, or gout.

Reliable sources for general information about nutrition, including menu planning and some recipes, may come from local health departments (which may have a Bureau of Nutrition), departments of nutrition at local community colleges and universities, local medical centers or societies, the American Heart Association, the American Diabetes Association, or the American Dietetic Association.

There are also many good cookbooks on the market that explain how to prepare meals that are simple, quick, and delicious. The U.S. Government Printing Office prints and sells general publications on nutrition. Single copies can be obtained free from the Consumer Information Center, Department 693-6, Pueblo, CO 81009.

Satisfying meals can be had when foods are whole, natural, and without sugar or chemicals. Then there is little reason to binge or cheat. Treat yourself to a natural foods cookbook. Among the best are Annemarie Colbin's *The Natural Gourmet* (Ballantine Books: N.Y., 1989) and Mary Estella's *Natural Foods Cookbook* (Japan Publications: N.Y., 1985).

FOOD BUDGET ASSISTANCE

Foods stamps are coupons that are provided by the government to use as cash in stores or for home-delivered meals. They help the elderly to defray some food costs by assuming part of the burden so that the recipients can afford to buy more nutritious food. Food-stamp eligibility is determined by income. Contact your local Department of Social Services to see if you qualify for food stamps.

Many older people are reluctant to use the services that the government has mandated as their entitlement. They recognize that these programs have been established for everyone; but because they grew up in a climate of self-reliance, it is difficult for them to admit that after working all of their lives they do not have sufficient income to feed themselves properly. Pride may thus act as a barrier to taking any financial assistance from the government, or even from children.

In these days, when most people are under economic pressure to make ends meet, anything that can help you stretch your food budget to include more nutritious items should be extremely welcome. The message is clear: man does not live by bread alone, but he cannot live without it. Help is available if you will but ask for it.

Regular Checkups

Our suggestions about the necessity for proper nutrition also apply to keeping healthy. Illness makes us feel wretched and exaggerates our woes. In addition, your patient will lose the benefit of your care and may become very upset and agitated by your illness and the concomitant changes in his daily routine. Do yourself a favor and see your doctor for regular checkups.

If you have recently had difficulty seeing things at a distance, or in very bright light, or if you've lost your ability to focus on near objects, your pleasure in reading, handwork, or walking outdoors will be inhibited, and your ability to do household tasks may be as well. Make sure that your glasses, if you wear them, have the correct prescription. Seeing ability declines as we get older.

When you have trouble understanding the dialogue of a TV program, or if you don't seem to be understanding what people say to you, it may be that your attention and concentration is not on the sound. If you can't hear a noise everyone else remarks upon, it's time to have your hearing checked. All of us lose part of the ability to hear high-pitched sounds as we get older and some sensory adequacy decreases. Some of us lose hearing ability a little sooner than others.

We have previously commented that good teeth and gums are important to eating a well-rounded diet. Have the dentist check yours regularly. Or, if you wear dentures, make sure that they continue to fit properly. This is especially important if you have recently lost a substantial amount of weight.

Illness Emergency Plans

Just as parents with small children generally have an emergency plan in case they become ill or have an accident, so must you have alternative solutions to protect yourself and your impaired relative if you should become ill or incapacitated.

Be sure you have established a network of supporters on whom you can call if something should happen. You may be able to rely on other members of your family, on people from your church or temple, or on professional health-care workers who are already involved in the care of your patient to step in if you become sick. Discuss with your friends and family in advance what would need to be handled if you were sick. It's much easier to recuperate if you don't have to worry about all the other aspects of your life.

Keep a notebook of emergency procedures where you write the telephone numbers of people who must be notified if a crisis occurs. It should have in it the number of your physician, pharmacist, nearest relative, and a reliable friend or neighbor. Make notes about your patient's medications and any peculiarities of behavior of which you are aware. Also note how specific things work (if unusual), such as the need to light the pilot on the stove in order to turn on the burners.

As a part of your planning, design an emergency alert system. You can use any of several aids: the emergency telephone number (generally 911) in your area; a walkie-talkie or intercom system that you share with a trusted friend, relative, or neighbor; an automatic dialing feature on your telephone that will alert local health or medical authorities to a crisis in your house; portable "panic buttons"; telephone reassurance systems, which offer regular (daily) check-ins by friends or volunteers; or a senior citizens' buddy system. Your emergency plan should consider the possibility that your relative, upset or confused by his perception of your illness, may panic and try to stop anyone from coming into your house to help you. He may obstruct life-saving procedures by locking the door and not letting paramedics in or by hiding the car keys. For this reason, make sure that one of the people whom you will alert in your emergency plan has copies of the keys to your house and your car.

If your illness involves a hospitalization, your relative must be cared for by others. You should make a plan for this possibility now, too, no matter how uncomfortable it makes you to think of your own illness and to plan for it. If you are facing nonemergency surgery or some other planned hospital stay, you will have time to arrange for respite care for your relative. When an emergency hospital stay is necessary, the person who is to look after your relative in your absence should be someone with whom he is familiar.

There are other alternatives: day care, temporary home health aide car, temporary institutionalization, senior centers, volunteer services, help from friends and neighbors, visiting nurse associations, and home health care agencies.

Use Medications with Care and Respect

As we grow older, the accumulated strains and injuries our bodies have suffered require more care and attention. Frequently, we use medications to relieve pain, regulate faulty body processes, and maintain a normal life. Medications must be handled with care and respect. It is important that you learn about medicines for your own health, safety, and sense of well-being. Here are some common guidelines for their use:[1]

1. When you tell your physician and your pharmacist about other medications you are taking, include not only prescription medicines but also those nonprescription preparations that you buy over the counter, such as antacids, aspirins, and laxatives.

1. Adapted from *Physicians' and Pharmacists' Guide to Your Medicines,* by the United States Pharmacopoeial Convention, Inc. (Ballantine Books: N.Y., 1981), p. viii.

2. Let your dentist know about any medicines you are taking before having dental surgery. (Of course, you should follow the same rule before any kind of surgery, but dental surgery frequently seems so minor—a shot of painkiller for a filling, perhaps—that we tend to overlook the possibility of synergistic reactions.)

3. Tell your doctor about any unusual or allergic reactions to medications.

4. Ask your pharmacist or doctor what the medicine contains, especially if you are on a special low-sugar, low-salt diet or are allergic to any substance.

5. Take your medication exactly as the doctor prescribed it. Use it for the full length of time unless you are otherwise instructed. Follow the directions on the label of a nonprescription drug.

6. Call your physician if you feel the medication is not working for you.

7. Store medicines in a cool, dry place such as a bathroom or kitchen cabinet. Keep medicines out of the reach of children and also out of sight of your memory-impaired relative. Don't put medicines in the refrigerator unless you are advised to do so by your doctor.

8. Store your medicines in their original containers. Leave the labels intact. Keep medicines tightly shut when not in use.

9. Never take or give medication in the dark.

10. Be aware of expiration dates on medications. Don't store medicines that are out-of-date, or use any over-the-counter medication that is more than one year old.

11. If you think you have overdosed on any medication, or if someone has taken medicine by accident, call your poison control center, physician, or pharmacist immediately. Keep those telephone numbers posted prominently near your telephone.

     Keep a bottle of Ipecac syrup stored safely in the bathroom cabinet. Use it if you are told to induce vomiting, but before you use it, be sure to read the directions on the label.

12. Check with your physician if you notice unusual reactions or side effects from a medication you are using.

13. Never give your medicine to another person. Each medicine is prescribed for a unique individual and his complaint. It may not be the appropriate treatment for someone else.

14. Know both the brand names and the generic names of medications you use. Generic medicines are cheaper. In some states, your pharmacist must (by law) give you the generic drug to fill your prescription if you ask for it.

15. Write down the names of medications you (or your relative) are taking. Also, write down questions to ask your doctor or pharmacists at the next visit, to make sure you get the desired information.

16. Don't wait until you are completely out of a medicine before you go to the pharmacy if you need a refill, especially if the medication is a vital one (such as nitroglycerin for heart patients). Before the prescription can be refilled, your pharmacist may be required to check with your doctor—that takes time! The pharmacy may have to order your medicine. If you give them enough time and advance warning, you will be the winner and won't have to wait.

Finally, as Fred Matlock has discovered, there are yet other actions you can take, both for your own better health and as a gift of love and concern for the person you are caring for:

"One day, after he had examined my wife, her doctor said to me, 'Fred, I want to examine you, too—and don't worry about the cost—this is "on the house." ' He gave me an examination, and then he asked me, 'Are you serious when you tell me how much you love your wife, or is it just a lot of bull?'

"I answered him, 'Yes! Look into my heart and you'll know how much I love her.' In 43 years I can't imagine any husband being happier than I was.

" 'Well, if that's the case,' he said, 'let me have your cigarettes.' He took my pack of cigarettes, crushed it, and threw it in the sink. Then he said, 'If you want to live to be able to take care of your wife, stop smoking, or you'll have emphysema six months from now.'

"I haven't had a cigarette since. I feel good about that for myself as well as for her."

CHAPTER 16

Exercises for a
Healthy Body

*W*e all need a break from our everyday lives. Working people take vacations. Parents who send their small children to a day care center generally find that both they and their children are refreshed by the few hours' respite from each other's company. Throughout our lives, family and community times must be balanced with moments of private revitalization and renewal.

As a caregiver to someone with Alzheimer's disease, your need for respite, refreshment, and privacy is as great as it ever was and may even have increased. At the same time, you may feel that the increased demands that are put on you by your patient's needs make it almost impossible for you to find time for recreation and release.

Nevertheless, relief is possible. It is also necessary, not only for you but for your impaired relative as well. Doing things for yourself and having time away from your patient will help you to function better.

The feeling of helplessness that you and other caregivers experience in the face of this illness is frightening and can become overpowering. The constant needs and demands of the impaired patient seem to encircle and threaten to engulf you. When you feel trapped in this way, unable to escape the situation, the terrible feelings of helplessness increase to the point where you may become overwhelmed.

This is the time to remember that being good to yourself and doing the best you can for your patient are not necessarily contradictory ideas. Only when you can do things for yourself that give you some sense of pleasure or respite from the twenty-four-hour-a-day, seven-day-a-week, fifty-two-week-a-year burden will you feel less helpless and thus be able to continue to give loving care to your relative.

Try to get away every day, even if it is only for an hour. After you have had a break, you will feel more competent and more in control of your life. With your self-confidence restored, you will once more be ready to cope with the unexpected setbacks that occur in daily life with a person who has Alzheimer's disease.

Mary Converse is a volunteer at the local library one morning a week. Her neighbor comes over to sit with her husband while she's out. "I don't know what I'd do without that half day!"

Phil Marquette works three and a half days a week—for his sanity, he says. "I have a bastard of a boss. But that's good, because I'm forced to—like a soldier—toe the line. It keeps me firm. I can't fall apart."

Georgina Bay sings in her church choir. "My voice isn't much good, but that doesn't really matter. I do it for myself! When I come home from choral practice, my husband always seems a little easier to handle. And when things get difficult, I can always look forward to singing Tuesday night and Sunday morning."

The Benefits of Exercise

Frustration, anger, depression, and stresses that come with caring for memory-impaired patients are reflected in our bodies as physical tension. We feel "tight," "cramped," or "jumpy." Exercise is perhaps one of the most important ways to reduce that physical tension. Relieving physical stress can help us manage our emotions more successfully. Relaxing the body by walking, climbing stairs, running, swimming, riding a bicycle, or doing light housework can increase physical energy and efficiency.

Exercise enables us to sleep more restfully and to awaken refreshed, to be fully alert throughout the day, and to feel more completely in control of ourselves and our lives. It can give us a general feeling of mental and physical well-being, which helps to lighten the weight of caregiving responsibilities that can literally and figuratively slump our shoulders. In addition, exercise helps us burn calories and maintain optimum body weight.

Would you like to be more vigorous, increase your body's work capacity, retard the aging of your nerve cells, help your heart deliver more oxygen to the tissues of your body, slow the loss of your muscle tissue, prevent your joints from wearing out, improve your appearance, expand your energy reserves, improve your circulation, and increase your range of arm and leg motion? Then exercise! So say the sports medicine physicians and physical fitness experts.

If you have never participated in active sports or cultivated a regular regimen of exercises and physical activity, you may be somewhat skeptical of the virtues ascribed to exercise by fitness enthusiasts. And, if your life has been for the most part sedentary, you may not realize what a remarkable difference regular and sustained physical exercise can make in your emotional state. The best way to see for yourself is to try it.

Walking

Walking for pleasure and exercise seems to be more of a European custom than an American one. Americans are great shoppers, so what walking they do tends to be more functional. Since walking is both an excellent exercise and one that is easily available to most of us, it is probably worthwhile for you to create for yourself opportunities to do additional walking. If there is a pretty park or seaside beach or boardwalk nearby, take a bus or drive the car to it, then get out and enjoy the surroundings on foot. Take your shoes off, if you wish, and luxuriate in the grass or sand beneath you; give your feet some freedom. When you walk with your memory-impaired relative, be careful that he does not walk on glass or shells that could cause blisters or bleeding.

291

Walking in the fresh air, even on a cold day, improves our breathing and stimulates the metabolism. The sun provides a natural source of vitamin D and helps to elevate our spirits. Walk a distance and then rest. You can increase the distance you walk each day.

After you have been walking for ten or fifteen minutes, you may become more aware of your surroundings. As you walk and begin to notice the trees, flowers, and birds, to nod to fellow walkers, and to smell the ocean air or the tantalizing whiff of a nearby barbecue, you may discover another benefit to be derived from exercise—the feeling that, at least for the moment, all's right with the world.

Strenuous Activity

Strenuous activity burns up excess energy and can help relieve tension. Caregivers use many activities to get exercise and "let off steam," such as scrubbing floors, walking at a pace of approximately four miles per hour for one hour, playing several sets of tennis (singles), swimming laps at a continuous pace, or dancing. Less strenuous activities include bowling, typing, doing light housework like mopping floors, vacuuming, or cleaning windows, and walking at approximately two miles per hour.

Tension-Relieving Exercises for Indoors

To give yourself a good feeling without having to take a trip to the country, try using tension-releasing exercises a few minutes each day. The following four exercises are simple to do:

1. Stand and stretch as high as you can reach. Then bend from the waist and hang. Let your arms hang loosely, and your head drop. Bounce gently ten times. While in this position, shake your head yes five times, then shake your head no five times. Straighten and stretch again.

2. Drop your chin on your chest. Slowly and gently rotate your head, putting your right ear on your right shoulder, then around and back to front position. Continue to rotate your head, putting your left ear on your left shoulder, then around and back, and finally returning your head to its original position. Do this three times in each direction. Several repetitions, always done slowly (never jerk your head), will relieve the tension in your neck.

3. Pull your shoulders back and rotate forward and back five times; then reverse, rotating backward and forward five times. You'll feel your back crack if you are supple.

4. Place your hand on the back of your neck. At the base of the skull there is an indentation. Press your fingers into that indentation and massage your neck and backbone as far down as you can reach. Another way to stretch and relax the back muscles can be almost as simple as lying on the floor or sitting straight in a chair. While lying on your back, or sitting, suck in your stomach until you feel the flat of your back against the floor or your chair. Then relax. Do this five times.

Treat yourself to an exercise book. Buy one that has pictures and simple directions, and follow some of the photographs. There are also videotapes available that you can borrow from the local library or buy at a video center if you have a VCR. If you are in doubt about beginning a program of exercises because you have never done them before or because you are not sure how much your body can safely do, ask your physician to arrange for an exercise stress test. The test is also available at hospital clinics, preventive medicine institutions, and at many YMCAs.

It is preferable to exercise in the morning, but noon, evening, or whenever you can is better than not at all. Try to do it at the same time each day, however, at a time when you're not expecting the phone or the doorbell to ring. Tell people you're not available during that specific time each day. Switch on lively music or get an exercise record and begin!

Warming Up

Before starting every workout, warm up with about ten minutes of calisthenics. Stretch the way you do when you're getting out of bed in the morning. Do it slowly, deliberately, languorously, like a cat. Allow your muscles to relax and "let go." Move slowly whenever you do a stretching exercise. Relax and breathe into the stretch.

After your warm-up, spend fifteen to twenty minutes split equally between walking and jogging (small running steps). Progress gradually to mostly jogging over a period of ten weeks. Do this at least three times a week. If it is too strenuous, don't jog, just walk rhythmically.

All you need is about forty minutes per session, several times a week. Following are some of the exercises you can include in your routine.

An Exercise Sampler

1. Kick off your shoes. Stand straight. Stretch your arms up to the ceiling as high as you can. Reach with your whole body. Stretch each arm higher than the other ten times. Then put both arms down. Start with three times, then increase to ten.

2. Bend at the waist. Stretch one arm out as if to swim, then the other. Do an overarm swimming motion. Start by facing straight ahead; ten facing front; ten facing right; ten facing left. (This exercise stretches arm and shoulder muscles and relieves tension.)

3. Shift your hips. Keep your knees straight, extend your arms out sideways, and shift your weight from side to side as far as possible. Get a good stretch. (This exercise trims hips and thighs and relieves lower back tension.) Start slowly; don't throw your hips. Do ten times.

4. Bend your knees halfway. Keep your heels on the floor, feet straight, and tuck your seat right under you. Tighten your buttocks and abdominal muscles and bend your knees. Then straighten up. Do ten times. (This exercise stretches the heel cords and strengthens feet and leg muscles.)

Exercises that increase your breathing and your heart rate also build stamina. To build stamina you have to work out every other day. Jogging, swimming, running, bicycling, or jumping increases endurance.

Sports like tennis increase endurance if you play hard enough. Stamina is the ability to keep going longer and helps you to have the energy to get through unexpected emergencies. Select other exercises for strengthening muscles and for flexibility and good posture. When you lift anything, do it correctly to ease your back. Never stand straight and pull. Always bend your knees and lift gradually.

When you sit down, lower yourself into a chair gradually and gracefully. When you are seated, sit up straight with your lower back flush against the back of the chair. Slumping in a chair can cause fatigue.

Bonnie Prudden, the 65-year-old head of the Institute for Physical Fitness in Stockbridge, Massachusetts, suggests the "ten-penny trick" as an indoor exercise. Put ten pennies on the floor and pick them up one by one and put them on a high shelf. Gradually increase the number of pennies. This exercise is good for the thigh muscles.

Another Bonnie Prudden exercise uses a "pet rock" weighing about one or two pounds. Keep the rock near the telephone. While you're talking on the phone, hold the weight in your free hand and swing it over your head, down to your side, up and around. Then switch hands.

COOLING DOWN

After your workout, cool down with ten to fifteen minutes of yoga-type stretching exercises. These are lighter exercises, and they will prevent joint and muscle injuries and heart problems. Relaxation acts as a way to cool off. While exercise stimulates, before bedtime it also prepares us for rest.

1. Sit on the floor with your legs crossed as much as you can. Rest your hands on your knees and let the head hang. Relax. Hold for one minute.

2. Lie on your back; draw your knees up to your chest. Close your eyes; breathe deeply. If your neck is tired or tense roll it slowly from side to side. This exercise helps to rest your back.

3. Finish your cool-down with a good stretch. Lie on your back (either on the floor or on a bed) with legs extended in front and your arms at your sides. Slowly stretch your right arm over your head and flex your right foot. Hold for a count of two. Then bring your arms back down and relax your foot. Repeat with the left foot and left arm. Relax.

4. Lie on your back and keep one knee bent to relax your back. Let go in all of your body.

5. Lie on your side and relax the knees.

6. Rest on your stomach, keeping one knee bent to relax the lower back.

Remember, the effects of exercise cannot be stored. Muscles must be toned every two or three days. Therefore, exercising should be done at least three nonconsecutive days a week, although exercising daily is ideal. To get the full benefit to the whole body, the minimum amount of exercise you should have in a day is twenty minutes. Exercise to music for maximum enjoyment.

CHAPTER 17

Exercises for a
Healthy Mind

As you watch, day after day, the instances and accumulated effects of memory loss in the life of someone you love, you may well wonder whether such a thing could happen to you. "How come I keep forgetting the name of my new next-door-neighbor?" "If I don't make a list of the three things I want at the store, I often forget one of them—am I losing my mind?" "Is there any way to keep my memory working?"

Most of us, as we grow older, experience the phenomenon of memory loss more often than we did when we were young. And we worry about it more than we used to. When a person of 30 or 35 forgets a name, a face, or the item on a grocery list, he's likely to say to himself, "Oh, well, it'll come back to me in a minute," while the person of 65 or older will wonder, "Am I losing my memory?"

The fact is, fewer than 10 percent of the older people in the United States suffer the catastrophic memory loss of Alzheimer's disease. All of us, however, experience a slowing-down in our mental processes, because the speed with which the aging nervous system is able to handle information decreases as one ages. Mild memory lapses are normal in many people at age 50. By age 60 we might experience slight changes in spatial perception and attention. When people are 70 years old, small changes in abstract thinking and language are considered normal. The deceleration may account for the differences in learning, memory, motor skills, and perception between older and younger people.

Primary memory refers to the ability to pick out a seven-digit telephone number from a directory and dial it from memory, an act that people in their sixties and seventies can perform as well as 20-year-olds. Secondary memory operates when, for example, you are shown a list of words and asked to repeat them. Older people don't recall as many words toward the middle of the list as younger people do. Therefore older people are less likely to retain "new" information and should have it presented to them more slowly.

Nevertheless, it is a myth that advancing age causes memory problems. Many other factors cause memory problems in both older and younger people: selective attention, lack of interest in what you are learning, distraction or simply not paying attention, and depression. Too much stress can disrupt the cognitive process: for example, some people completely forget the material they have learned when they are tested in an examination. Frequent social drinking weakens memory; heavy drinking obliterates it.

Memory is like a muscle. All muscles must be exercised if they are to retain their tone. The same is true of your memory—use it or lose it. Actually, memory is a set of activities and skills that dictate what we do with information. If we process and store information inefficiently, we'll have difficulty in the retrieving process.

Some memory loss is a function of environmental change. You may know your psychotherapist's name perfectly well in the office, but draw a blank when the two of you meet at the supermarket.

As we acquire more knowledge, new and old memories compete with one another, sometimes causing interference. (Did you ever reach for the emergency brake where it used to be in your old car?)

There are times when forgetfulness is useful. It may help us to keep our memories from becoming overloaded. It also helps to ease the pain of growing older in a society that venerates youth. Yet we remain capable of learning throughout life—provided we are sufficiently stimulated and challenged. Mild stress can even improve memory, by forcing the brain to produce chemical stimulants that increase mental efficiency.

Keeping Memory "In Shape"

Although we may forget the names of people we know or where we put our glasses, these memory lapses are a normal part of living. Memory lapses occur at all ages. For youths these are amusing moments; for older people they can be embarrassing or frightening reminders that old age causes memory loss. With motivation and practice, memory lapses can be helped by good habits such as orderliness, planning, organization, and the use of memory aids—appointment books, calendars, notes on the refrigerator door, a wristwatch timer, a kitchen timer. Writing lists, organized by categories, or putting things back in the same place each time is also helpful.

Your attitude about remembering is extremely important. Not everything has to be remembered; you also can't remember things you've never learned or have not made part of your conscious awareness. For example, if you are thinking about something else while you are reading the newspaper, you won't remember what you've read because other thoughts have been interfering. The enjoyment of the activity itself—reading, attending movies, watching television—should take priority over remembering specific content. But if you do want to remember the content, tell someone about what you saw or read, make notes about it, and try to form some associations and connections to the material you want to remember. Your ability to remember will be enhanced by three key memory skills: concentration, association, and repetition.

Try new approaches and strategies in each area of your life. Don't worry that a forgotten phone number or book title means that you're a candidate for Alzheimer's disease. Remember, if you're preoccupied or depressed, you will tend to be more forgetful. Take forgetting in your stride and be patient and compassionate with yourself. You will probably remember the item when you least expect to, and you will also tend to recall what is most important to you.

There are some helpful principles and techniques that can make our memories more useful and efficient.[1]

1. Adapted from Z. Goldberg, et al., *The Wadsworth Memory Enhancement Program for Older Adults.* (Los Angeles: Neurology Service, V.A. Wadsworth Medical Center, 1980). Used with permission.

1. Pay attention. If you didn't consciously notice where you put your umbrella or where you parked your car, you won't remember. Such failure to pay attention is a form of absentmindedness. Instruct yourself as you put down your glasses: "I am putting my glasses on the desk." By focusing your attention on what you're doing, you reduce the possibility of walking off and forgetting your glasses. As you do the task, verbalize it. When you turn off the gas, say to yourself: "I have turned off the gas jets."

2. Use physical reminders to capture your own attention. Just as advertisers use bright colors, flashing lights, or surprising turns of phrase to capture our attention, so we may gain our own attention by the obvious or the unusual. Wear a rubber band around your wrist (or tie a string around your finger) to remind you of something. Set the laundry in front of the door on the day you plan to take it to the laundromat.

3. To remember a person's name, make a special effort to attend to his name as he gives it. Look directly at him and make eye contact. Then rely on association—convert the verbal into something visual. Pick out the person's most noticeable facial feature and merge it with a ridiculous word-picture of the name. For example, if you are introduced to Mr. Meistersinger, and he has bushy eyebrows, you could visualize using a spoon to stir his eyebrows ("Me stir man's eyebrow").

   Make sure you hear the person's name as well; repeat it. Focus on the name: is it funny, unusual, common? Does it fit the person? Try to remark about it. Use the name several times in conversation or in a question. All these devices help you to remember it.

4. Organization is effective in helping to retrieve information from your memory. Therefore, try to group pieces of information together. For example, if you're trying to remember a telephone number, make chunks of the digits, two or three at a time—that is, for the number 873-2132, remember 873, then 21, then 32, in separate groups. Don't try to remember each number individually.

   Use cues to remember to do certain things at certain times—for example, remember that you always leave for work after you hear the 8:00 AM news.

Make lists. Writing things down is a positive habit. Taking notes actually improves the memory because doing so makes you an active learner. When you make a list, arrange the items in categories. Say you have nine grocery items: tissues, bread, milk, cheese, paper napkins, toilet tissue, chicken, steak, cream, and butter. Group the items into four dairy, two meat, three paper products, and so on. Use your lists to remember things you want to do or want to tell someone.

Use all the devices you can think of when you are presented with new material in order to try to instill it firmly in your memory. We remember something best when we have learned it well in the first place.

There is no need for panic if you don't remember a name, a face, or a task. Be patient, it will come to you later.

Finally, don't demand too much of yourself. You cannot be expected to remember what you have never learned.

Can Foods Improve Memory?

Very little is known about the effect of nutrition on brain function. While large doses of lecithin and choline have been used experimentally in treating patients with Alzheimer's disease, there is no conclusive evidence that these nutrients can reverse or stop the process of memory loss. Choline, found in foods such as liver, egg yolks, soybeans, wheat germ, lecithin, and peanuts, is absorbed directly from the bloodstream by the brain. There it is converted to acetylcholine, the neurotransmitter (an electrochemical substance) that carries nerve impulses across the synapse and stimulates neurons to send signals from the brain to other cells.

Research indicates that people with severe memory loss have a deficiency of acetylcholine in their brains. However, the amount of such chemical (or nutrient, for nutrients are chemicals) that is necessary to affect the brain is so great that it would be impossible to use food to obtain the same effect or impact. At some time in the future, administering pure sources of acetylcholine might prove helpful in treating memory impairment.

At the present time, the emphasis in nutrition is on preventing health problems, rather than on curing ones that already exist. As far as we know, there appear to be no special foods or diets that can improve memory impairment.

Become Your Own Nurturer

We all have varying degrees of "personality hardiness," that is, the ability to cope with life's ups and downs. If you have a clear sense of identity and know who you are, you can look at the inevitable tensions of life as challenges rather than threats. By acquiring compassion and love for ourselves, we can learn to lick our own wounds, temper our desires, tolerate our weaknesses, and exercise self-discipline, always remembering that a temporary lapse in self-control does not mean that we are failures.

Try to soothe yourself. Instead of feeling defeated, we can pick ourselves up and try, try again, without blaming or punishing ourselves for inevitably falling off the straight and narrow. With a conviction that our lives are purposeful, we can pursue love and achieve our goals.

Reason with yourself. Know that rejection is part of living and not necessarily something that happens because we're undeserving or because we've done something to earn it.

Overcome insecurity and practice positive self-regard. Does this mean be thoughtless, mean, and selfish? No way. It means you have sufficient self-respect to care about and for yourself—your own health and your happiness.

Give yourself enough time to do what you need and want to do. Ask yourself, what's meaningful to me? Arrange your daily schedule so that you have time to do something personally satisfying and gratifying each day. You'll be in much better shape to tend to the needs of your family, friends, and patients after you've done your own thing. You won't feel put upon or resentful if you have enough time for yourself.

Let others know who you really are. If you're frightened, anxious, tense, or nervous about something, tell someone. Letting others know about it allows them to know you as you really are without pretense. It takes courage to reveal our fears or anxieties, but once revealed, you'll have a vast sense of inner peace. Few individuals can cope with trauma or crisis alone. We need each other's support during stressful times, especially when fears of illness and feelings of helplessness or hopelessness invade our thoughts. Reach out to friends and to strangers with love and caring. It will help you become self-assured.

Rely on yourself. It will empower you. Learning to do things by and for yourself frees you from feelings of vulnerability. Taking care of mechanical things and finances are things women usually leave to men because they don't want to take the time and trouble to learn about them. Remember, if you rely on someone else (a man or a woman) to give you all that you desire, that person also has the power to take it away. Doing things we don't necessarily like to do helps to keep us in balance. Ultimately, mastery makes us feel stronger, more competent, and self-reliant.

Plan work that is creative and engrossing. All creative endeavors require periods of being alone, free from the distractions and noises of other people. In order for life to be a creative process, each of us independently must find our own creative source. When we locate our creative energies, we can allow them to flow through our lives. In that way we will leave an imprint on whatever we do. Simply do your best in your own unique way. Your uniquely creative way is what gives meaning to your life.

Make yourself an offer you can't refuse. Focus on becoming a trusting, responsible, highly motivated, and committed person to yourself. Only make promises to yourself when your goals are realistic and achievable. Keeping a promise may mean being tough on yourself and less permissive than before. Saving money or following a diet or an exercise program are contracts we can make with ourselves. Keeping the contract may entail a sacrifice (no new blouse for a month, a taboo on chocolate, or doing the Jane Fonda tape daily). But fulfilling the contract also means more self-esteem, increased strength, more personal satisfaction, and joy.

After you've done this, evaluate the plan as it is in progress: follow as planned—change the steps or add other resources—then celebrate your newly found courage and accomplishments!

Think positively about yourself. Build your self-esteem by letting yourself know that you are a fine person with good instincts and warm feelings toward yourself and others. Successful people believe that failure is just an obstacle on the pathway to success. Dream of success and have a passion to succeed in this world. Your determination will give you the will and energy to accomplish your goals. Believe in yourself; know that your time will come and that failure is impossible.

Trust Yourself to Have Self-Control

Underlying our struggle to grow into healthy, mature, responsible people is the common thread of having to provide nurturance, protection, comfort, and soothing to ourselves just as it was (hopefully) provided for us in our infancy. To do this we need the inner resilience that helps us to master our bodies and our minds. Awareness helps us to trust ourselves and to have self-control. Our internal feeling of being in control of ourselves tends to reduce negative emotions. It stimulates effort, involvement, and the ability to cope with difficult problems. Therefore, it is essential that we have a daily routine with purposeful, tangible reminders that we are in charge of ourselves and our future.

We may not always be able to control outer reality (the environment), but we can be in control of our own inner reality—our thoughts, wishes, ideas, feelings, our values, our needs, and even our own dreams. Self-control enhances our self-confidence and activates internal feelings of being worthwhile and having value as individuals.

Have a clear conscience. Avoid the traps of self-recrimination, and shed the mantles of guilt. Don't blame yourself for your predicaments. Get on with your life with a constructive force of energy. Through joyful and zestful living you'll resolve old hurts, work through guilt and ambivalent feelings, and uplift your depression.

The test of maturity and confidence is to be able to distinguish good from bad stress and to develop practical coping skills that are useful and work in real life. The secret is to risk and try new experiences that can be rewarding. They'll help you to grow intellectually, emotionally, and spiritually.

Learn to enjoy being alone by using your imagination. Don't depend on the constant companionship of others. You'll feel more secure when you enjoy your own company. Then you can put people into your world through your imagination, or you can imagine yourself in a place you'd like to be. For example, imagine yourself now at a beautiful beach or on a cool mountaintop. Think how safe and comfortable you feel there. Focus on positive and healing thoughts and images in order to overcome negative and painful ones. Tell yourself you're feeling calm, happy, re-laxed. You're where you want to be, and so let go of all the tension that binds you. Unlock the tightness in your jaw, feel the bones in your neck begin to separate as you yawn, and relax the tension in the back of your neck and throughout your spine. Let all the tension go out through your fingers and down into the toes and out onto the pavement under your feet. Then picture yourself having a stimulating conversation with the next person who comes along—your friend, parent, sibling, or mate. Speak your mind openly, honestly, and assertively.

Lighten up. Let your sense of humor carry the day. Even a patient with Alzheimer's disease can joke about it. One woman quipped, "I would have to have this Wizenheimer's disease!" Humor can reframe our real-ity, and laughter can help people make a positive connection with each other.

Continue to Learn throughout Life

Continual learning throughout life adds to our capacities to derive meaning from life. In Chapter 10, we encouraged you to keep your memory-impaired relative active in the sports and hobbies he enjoyed in the past for as long as he is able to enjoy them. Now, what about you? Have you followed the same plan of action for yourself?

Do you still belong to the golf club? How is your garden this year? If you and your spouse used to play bridge together, do you still play? If your partner can no longer play, have you joined a "singles" league? How long has it been since you sat down for an hour with your weaving, woodworking, or needlecraft project?

You *can* find the time to pursue your own hobbies and interests. Your mind and spirit will benefit from the stimulation and variety. Arranging opportunities may not always be easy, but Ms. Kosciusko, who has been a caregiver for eight years, is convinced it is worthwhile:

> "You can wallow in self-pity when you have this burden, become stupefied, and stop growing and learning. But if you are determined to keep doing the things that you like to do, you can. It's a hard job, but do it! Read a book, see things, take a trip, go out to eat, do as much as you can. Many high schools and colleges have very inexpensive musical performances, so if you like music, go to concerts, go to the opera. Don't stop! I take my sister with me to all these things. She still enjoys music, and both of us feel better for the break."

For Ms. Kosciusko, sharing her pleasures with her sister is part of the enjoyment. Other caregivers want to pursue interests that are entirely separate from the lives they share with their impaired relatives.

> MRS. LILA BELLINGHAM: "I never worked in my entire life until my husband developed Alzheimer's disease. Now I can't stand to be around him all the time—his babbling infuriates me. I had always done needle-work for the church, so when the owner of our crafts shop asked me to work in her store, I jumped at the chance. I sell supplies and give lessons three days a week. I make about as much money as I pay the home health aide to stay with Charley, but I'd do it if it cost twice as much as I make."

Whatever your interests are, whether it's learning to speak French, playing cribbage, practicing a new piece of music, or growing orchids, your life will be enriched as you pursue hobbies, interests, and education.

Courses in art, music, politics, macrame, bridge, dancing, investments, and other subjects are offered at local high schools, colleges, senior citizens' centers, and centers for lifelong learning (often affiliated with a college, university, or national union). Rural areas offer courses through the Farm Bureau or Agricultural Extension Services or through agricultural and technical colleges.

Selecting a subject you have always wanted to study but didn't have time to pursue can be very rewarding. Returning to the study of a once-favorite hobby or subject is equally enjoyable and may bring a heightened sense of accomplishment.

Choosing to study in a classroom environment has the added advantage of meeting other people who share your interests. Some weekly bridge-playing afternoons and musical evenings have evolved from such courses. Concentrating on something outside of yourself and the opportunity of befriending new people are the additional benefits of such courses.

Your mental stimulation and interest in the topics you are studying may indirectly help your impaired relative. One woman told us that, as her father's illness reduced his ability to respond intellectually, his emotional sensitivity and responsiveness increased. He could always sense how other members of the family felt—whether they were happy, sad, discontented, annoyed, satisfied, cheerful, or blue—and his own reactions reflected their emotional state. If you are satisfied with yourself and feeling positive about what you are doing, it is possible that your relative will sense and in some way benefit from these good feelings, too.

But how will you manage to get away from the house long enough to study anything? The desire to do it is the first step. You may be able to arrange for a friend or relative to sit with your patient for just one morning, afternoon, or evening a week. Or, you might know someone from your support group who also wants to take a course on a different day with whom you could organize a joint caretaking arrangement. If the course you wish to take is at a senior citizens' center, there may be a day care program as a part of the center's activities where you can leave your relative while you go to class. There are probably many ways to solve this practical problem, but you yourself must be eager for a solution before you will find the time, energy, and initiative to explore the issue.

Maintain Your Spiritual Beliefs

The spiritual and religious side of our psyches can be the source of great comfort in trying times. A spiritual belief (whether focused on God, Christ, Allah, Buddha, or another center beyond specific social expression) is an inner belief. It transcends the material world. Satisfying inner beliefs can be developed through meditation and study, prayer, such rituals as burning incense, or whatever works for you.

Many philosophies of life, including those of Spinoza, Plato, and Tao, suggest that the universe contains all the power and information the body needs to get well. Carl Jung, a noted psychoanalyst and contemporary of Freud, philosophized that everything comes together in the universe: if you want to know what is right, you must also know what is wrong. If you want light, you must also have shadow, and if you want to know health, you must also know illness. Evidence from the disciplines of physics and psychology gives rise to the idea of a power behind the scenes that will stop at nothing to give us health. If we attune ourselves—surrender to the uncontrollable and "be" in a certain way—healing will manifest itself.

It requires trust to give up a sense of control in favor of faith in a higher wisdom. You must acknowledge that you may not be able to fully interpret the outcome of life. Your relative with Alzheimer's disease may become worse and die, and you may never understand why he developed the disease. We have to accept where the patient is in his life and what lessons we can learn from adversity. If we are open and receptive, we can find wisdom in whatever difficult moments life may offer us.

Use the Power of Your Imagination

Turn to your imagination to soothe yourself. You can change your negative emotions into positive emotions and create more positive attitudes towards newer and more creative life experiences.

Bolstering our ability to imagine ourselves in situations where we are able to cope with stress, depression, sleeplessness, anxiety, worry, and destructive behaviors can also improve our immune systems.

In turn, daily positive "coping imagery" can influence our physical and mental wellness. Each of the following exercises takes about fifteen minutes. Start with one or two, and then gradually incorporate them within a week's time into your daily routine. After you've done a coping image, bring yourself back to your surroundings by counting from one to five. Slowly orient yourself to your surroundings before taking up your usual activities

Breathe away stress to relieve minor health problems such as headaches, stomach aches, and skin disorders that may be rooted in stress. Here's how it works. Loosen any tight belts, scarves or other clothing that hampers relaxation. Be seated in a comfortable chair. Take a deep breath, hold it for five seconds, and then let it out slowly. When you let go, make a slight hissing sound. Take another deep breath and hold it again. Do this three times. (The new oxygen you're breathing in may make you feel a little lightheaded or dizzy. It will pass.) As you inhale, tell yourself "I am relaxed" and on the exhale say "relaxed." Do this several times, and as you exhale sink into the chair in which you're seated. Feel yourself becoming relaxed, slowing down. Feel the tension in your body slowing down and your mind slowing down. Breathe in the glow of relaxation, and breathe out fatigue, frustration, and tension. Feel at ease, at peace, with all that surrounds you.

Reliving happy memories can help to heal memories that are hurtful and that cause feelings of depression. Focusing on past events that were unpleasant can make us feel pessimistic. Positive thinking, optimism, and feelings of hopefulness can produce physiological changes in our immune systems that make us feel happier, give us increased strength to accomplish our goals, and keep us healthy.

Do this exercise in the morning upon waking and at night before going to bed. Breathe deeply, hold for ten seconds, then let go. Filter out the noises or chatter in your head.

Visualize your happiest moment—graduating from nursing school, your wedding, the birth of your first child, or some recognition of your achievements by a beloved person. Visualize a scene in which you felt someone's kindness, compassion, and love. Visualize yourself feeling kind or considerate, elated, or successful. Reexperience the events. Relive the joyful feelings. Dwell on the images—imprint them on your recent memory. Remember these wonderful feelings!

Resist insomnia by thinking of situations that make you feel very sleepy, such as staying up all night to study for an exam, or preparing for a lecture, or waiting for someone's plane or train to come in at 3:00 AM, or moonlighting by sitting up with a sick patient at night after working an eight-hour day shift. Concentrate on the image and disregard the demands of reality. Allow yourself to drift into sleep.

White-out your worries by imagining a great white ball of warming light covering your head and body. The light is inside your body and mind, dissolving negative thoughts and emotions. They go up in smoke and leave you feeling cleansed and free from care. What a joy!

Picture yourself shrinking away your viruses, colds, headaches, and wounds by imagining the body cavity involved. Then imagine yourself drawing the image of the wound or virus on a blackboard that needs to be erased. Erase the unhealthy picture and replace it with images of healthy cells or cleansing blood. Concentrate on focusing on the area that is sick. Imagine it to be well. Continue to practice this until you sense that you are healing.

Resist the temptation to continue destructive eating patterns, smoking and drinking alcohol, or taking drugs. Imagine yourself in each of these situations; as you are being tempted, a voice from within says, "Stop, listen, I don't need this anymore—I'm free." Then picture yourself thin, walking five miles, sober, rational. If you imagine that you haven't heeded the voice, imagine yourself fatter, drunk, bottomed out, or having emphysema. Practice resisting temptations several times a day.

Be in tune with your inner self. Close your eyes and imagine yourself on a mountaintop communing with a wise and compassionate advisor (a prophet, or perhaps, God). Talk to this person about your dilemmas. This person knows you well and may advise you. Hold onto the advice. When you are awake and fully alert, think about the advice, evaluate it, and if it seems to make sense and there is little risk involved, follow the advice. (In all probability, you are giving yourself good advice based on previous unconscious thoughts about your problems.)

As you have already gleaned from the pages you've read, being your own nurturer or mother or nurse, if you will, requires attentiveness and vigilance to your own needs. This is attained by a continuous struggle with yourself, since nurturance is a feeling from within. The huge reward that one gets is in the payoff—*freedom* to be who and what you want to be, which helps you to feel good about yourself. Your self-knowledge gives you the power to feel stronger and more confident, both personally and professionally.

When we ask, what does it all mean, we are journeying onto the path of what makes us human.

CHAPTER 18

Help for Troubled Caregivers

Alzheimer's disease is a family problem. The effects of the illness touch every member, even if only one person is the principal caregiver. Often, when that caregiver is the spouse, the caregiving role comes at a time when he or she is older and perhaps in poor health.

Many times, of course, children will become involved in a parent's care as well. For example, when an aging parent has lost a spouse, middle-aged daughters are most likely to take on the responsibility of daily care. Even when both parents are alive and one spouse might reasonably expect to care for the other, daughters often play an ancillary role in helping the caregiving parent to contact outside sources of help. When the parent feels unable to cope with the burden of an aging, confused spouse alone, female children and other female relatives often take over and assist in giving care. Perhaps this happens because females are raised to be nurturing and have traditionally been at home. They also tend to keep more closely in touch with their parents than males do. Even daughters-in-law who have good relationships with their parents-in-law take on the caregiver's role.

In our experience, males are likely to be primary caregivers either when they are "only" children or when a daughter has had an unhappy relationship with the parents and refuses the role of caregiver. Perhaps as women become more involved with careers outside the home, and domestic tasks are divided more evenly between men and women, more men will assume major caregiving responsibilities.

Sometimes a particular adult child is singled out as the person on whom the parents prefer to rely. Whether married or single, this is the child who can be counted on, who keeps closely in touch with the parents. Sometimes, one child may volunteer for the job, either unconsciously hoping to gain recognition and approval from others or responding to the feelings of guilt, because he feels he has received much more from his parents than the other siblings in the family. Adult children who have strong mutual bonds of affection with their parents make many sacrifices in order to ease their parents' lives.

Sometimes children become caregivers to their parents for reasons that are rarely apparent to themselves or to others but may be understood with the help of counseling. A child may, for example, become a "pseudocaregiver" who assumes the responsibility in name only but delegates his authority and the real work of caregiving to others. His own need to appear to be firmly ensconced in the affections of his parents (or perhaps his need to be a major beneficiary of their will) may be the principal motivation. The need for admiration from others may also contribute to this child's assuming such a role. Brothers and sisters may be aware of their sibling's motivation but often let him get away with it in order to preserve the status quo. Exposure would mean pain to the parent who needs his help.

The caregiver who insists on acting like a martyr by assuming the total burden of the relative's care is motivated by complex feelings toward his parents. Typically, this child discourages other family members from helping by his zealousness for the task, then later feels overburdened and complains of the personal discomfort resulting from the impossible demands he has placed on himself. If caregiving is the responsibility of such a child, the sick person may be used as a pawn in the family power struggle.

Those children who criticize each other at a distance and vie for the favorite position with parents, and those relatives who create dissension because of jealousy or conflicting loyalties, often contribute, deliberately or inadvertently, to increased tension and resentment in the family. When parental ties can no longer keep the family together, the wounds given and received during the illness of a parent may lead to the breaking of bonds between siblings, who may then never be reconciled.

No matter what the specific circumstances may be, children who must assume the care of a memory-impaired parent do so with reluctance and with real sorrow for the parent's loss of power and independence.

Becoming a Parent to Your Parent

Erich Garbino brought his 94-year-old grandfather to see a counselor, who was both a gerontologist and a psychotherapist, for an evaluation of the senior Mr. Garbino's ability to continue to live alone. Erich lived in the suburbs and found himself terribly uneasy if he couldn't reach his grandfather by telephone. Either Erich or his wife would telephone Mr. Garbino twice a day to make sure he was all right. One day, Mr. Garbino's telephone was off the hook. Erich tried to contact some friends who lived close to his grandfather, intending to ask them to look in on him. Finally, he became too anxious to wait and drove the eighty miles to his grandfather's house.

When he arrived, he found his grandfather in good health and spirits. Apparently his grandfather had neglected to put the receiver back on the hook after the previous night's telephone call. Much relieved, Erich drove home but decided it was time to see the counselor once again, as he had a few months earlier, for help in setting up the system of telephone calls and the network of friends that had enabled his grandfather to continue to live alone.

He explained to the counselor that his grandfather had become increasingly forgetful and had misplaced his house keys just a few days before. Also, a week before, Mr. Garbino had accused Erich of stealing his money. Erich was so devastated by his grandfather's accusation that he felt as if he had been kicked in the stomach.

As he spoke, it became clear that Erich, now 58, was a devoted grandson who had done everything in his power to help his widowed and elderly grandfather in the quarter-century since his grandmother's death. He treated his grandfather with respect and kindness.

A fiercely independent man, accustomed to taking care of himself, Mr. Garbino appeared healthy, clear, and well-dressed. His conversation was clear, except that whenever he couldn't remember or answer a question, he would say, "I'll have to look that up." Although he recognized that he sometimes needed "a little help," he was unwilling to give up his independence and wished to be responsible for himself as he has been "since I was a boy of seven."

Several ideas emerged from the conversation:

1. Erich's inability to take over the caregiving role was a result not only of his grandfather's tenacity in retaining his independence, but also of Erich's own need for approval from his grandfather. Going against his grandfather's wishes to remain independent would be, for Erich, a breach of faith that would trigger his grandfather's displeasure.

2. Mr. Garbino was a very strong-willed man who held on to his independence but did welcome assistance from his grandson and granddaughter-in-law.

3. Mr. Garbino was suffering from some memory failure and, despite his cleverness in concealing it, appeared to have declined in the several months since the first consultation. He would soon be unable to live independently.

Now the options were narrowing. Erich would have to work out his feelings about still wanting to be his grandfather's "good little boy who has Granddad's approval" with his own therapist. But in the interim, he would have to act like his grandfather's father and reverse roles with him. Despite his sadness and feelings of being overwhelmed, he would have to take over family leadership and certain responsibilities, such as finances. He would have to develop a safe, failproof system to protect his grandfather, regardless of the elder Garbino's disapproval of such arrangements.

At the same time, Erich and his wife would begin to investigate nursing homes, in the event that Mr. Garbino continued to deteriorate. The gerontologist would be available for further consultation when and if it became necessary. Erich left the counselor's office feeling reassured that he was doing the best he could for his grandfather. Mr. Garbino openly agreed to accompany Erich to see his cousin, an attorney, to "get his estate straightened out."

Jessica Humphreys, at the age of 28, took over the role of mothering her own mother when Sarah Humphreys had a stroke that left her paralyzed on one side of her body. Unable to speak, at the age of 63, Sarah remained able to communicate by writing notes. Jessica, the youngest of four children and the only unmarried daughter, felt it was her responsibility to arrange for a home health aide to take care of her mother while her retired father took over chores such as shopping, cooking, and tending to his wife's physical needs.

Unfortunately, he was not consistent and would sometime let Sarah stay in soiled sheets and clothing for a day or two. When Jessica realized that her father could no longer take care of her mother because of his own failing memory, she grudgingly accepted the reality and decided it was time for both of her parents to be placed in a nursing home. In her customary outwardly cool manner, Jessica began the long search for a suitable nursing home when her parents could share a room together.

It wasn't easy to find, but after several months, and with the support of her psychotherapy group, she was able to accomplish her goal. During her search, she would reveal to her group how intimidated she was by the social workers at each of the homes, and how worried she was about taking over her parents' finances. Behind all of her panic was the dread of making the wrong decision in the eyes of her brothers and sisters, and her fantasy that if her father recovered his memory or if her mother could talk, they would berate her for being a "bad little girl" because she didn't quit her job in order to stay home and take care of them. She felt guilty about being competent at work and about her unwillingness to shoulder the full burden of care of both her parents.

Yet she "parented" her parents remarkably well as she worked through her guilt about taking over and her uneasy feelings about being a responsible adult, something her mother had convinced her she would never really be. "You'll always be my baby," Jessica was told, from the time she would walk until she moved out of her parents' home at the age of 26 to begin an independent life. Secretly, Jessica believed her mother and did indeed feel like a baby walking around in an adult's body and clothing.

In both cases, having to reverse roles with their parents was very difficult for these adult children. It meant taking over as head of the household. They still felt as if they were themselves children, in need of their parents' approval in order to function independently.

Role reversal also means taking charge of your relative's medical care:

MR. DAVID CLIPPEN: "I'm sure that my father's hearing has become worse in the last few months. But I cannot get him to go to a doctor and have his hearing checked. It's so frustrating. It may be simply the result of aging, or a nerve deafness, or something like that which can't be helped, but it could be a blockage of some kind. It could be curable, or at least improvable. Some diseases are treatable if you catch them early. I would hate to have him go to an ear specialist two years from now and learn that we could have done something if we'd acted immediately.

"Every time I suggest to him that he should go to a doctor, he says, 'Why? Are you a bounty hunter for doctors? Do you get a reward every time you bring in a new victim?' Of course, what irritates me is that he is making a decision about his own condition without benefit of medical advice. He's probably saying to himself, 'I'm 89 years old, what can they do for me?' which is the wrong way to make a decision . . . and at the same time, maybe he's right.

"Meanwhile, I'm terribly frustrated by his refusal to see a doctor and frightened by the possibility that the deafness could represent something serious. I'm responsible for his health, in a certain way, and he makes it impossible for me to carry out that responsibility."

For spouses, changes in role may entail becoming a mother or father to your wife or husband. Since spouses frequently act as a loving mother or father to one another in times of uncertainty, and especially in time of illness, they are more accustomed to taking on some of the characteristics of that role. However, for some wives, parenting a husband may mean taking over a business, or the checkbook, and handling matters with which they've have no previous experience. For a husband, it may mean taking over household chores that never interested him and that he doesn't know how to do.

MR. GEORGE HILLERSON: "It's much more difficult for a man when his wife develops Alzheimer's disease, I think, than it is for a woman whose husband is ill. After all, she has always done all the nursing and the cooking and all that. The husband has to change his whole outlook. My wife prepared everything, took care of the home, did the wash, did everything, and all of a sudden the roles are completely reversed. My wife may have had problems of her own when I was sick, handling the finances and so on, but she didn't have to learn how to cook or how to shop. I never knew the price of an egg. Now I can tell you what every supermarket's got. I'm really getting an education. I never showed an interest. I didn't care. Now I must see to it that there's milk and bread in the house and that the refrigerator is full. I never realized what a big job homemaking is, and I used to wonder what my wife did all day—now I know!"

Husbands and wives usually take responsibility for each other and manage to stay together "in sickness and in health until death us do part." Some have described themselves as "prisoners of love." What makes any couple try to contribute to the happiness of each other and to experience both the good and the bad times together? Many spouses ask theoretically, "Wouldn't he take care of me in the same way if I were sick?" Genuine empathy for the other person and the ability to understand develops over many years. These feelings are linked with equally strong feelings of responsibility and concern.

It is only fair to point out, however, that these are not universal feelings. There are also those husbands and wives who have not had a good relationship with their spouses but who have remained in the marriage for various reasons: "because of the children," or "because I didn't have any place to go," or "because I was too weak to walk out." These are the unwilling caregivers. For them, the responsibility of caring for a memory-impaired spouse at home looms large. There is added resentment about the wasted years of the past and those of the future, when the caregiver will confront the prospect of living alone after the spouse has been placed in an institution.

> Ms. ANNETTE YORIPOLSKI: "You say to yourself, 'After what we've been through, I don't owe this guy a thing!' And then you recount to yourself the reasons you don't owe him, and you get more and more resentful of the fact that you have to care for him day after day and night after night. Now, maybe if we'd had a more comfortable married relationship, it might not be that way. He was so selfish that I have no guilt feelings at all. I know that without me, no one would care enough to take care of him.
>
> "Well, maybe I feel a little guilty about the fact that I'm not actually with him 24 hours a day—I have a woman who comes in to take care of him while I'm at work—because I think it would be good for him if I were there. But by the same token, I know I couldn't survive it. And I must survive, because he has no one else to care for him but me."

In addition to the emotional responsibility that husbands and wives feel for each other, they are also, unlike children, legally responsible for each other financially, as we noted in Chapter 13. This situation leads many spouses, whether they are rich or poor, to refuse to place the failing partner in a nursing home, even when it becomes necessary. This resistance is often damaging to the unimpaired spouse, who becomes physically and mentally exhausted trying to care for his or her partner at home.

Christopher Dressler tried to keep his wife at home out of his own sense of dependency on her and his need to take care of her—and also because of his miserliness. He was reluctant to spend the money that nursing home placement would require ($3,600 per month), fearing that he would be left penniless, despite the fact that he had already put most of their money in a trust fund in his son's name.

He hesitated even to hire a home attendant: "I don't want anyone around and underfoot," he argued. "Besides," he reassured himself, "she can still be left alone without being a danger to herself." Yet, every time Mr. Dressler returned home, he found his wife, Virginia, bewildered, angry, or not knowing who he was. He fought with her, sometimes shouting at her, occasionally shaking her, until the stress propelled him to have a heart attack.

Now, as he lies in the hospital recuperating, in essence his problems with Virginia are solved. But surely his own troubles now begin as he faces bypass surgery, the long period of recovery, bed rest, and eventual reorganization of his fast-paced and somewhat frenetic life. Did he need to have a heart attack to say to his son and family, "I need a rest. I need help. This is a serious problem for me with which I can't cope. I feel helpless and desperate!"

Perhaps now Mr. Dressler will be able to come to terms with some of those feelings of helplessness. Then, with the cooperation of his son and family, he may be able to care for his wife without destroying himself.

How Families Can Resolve Issues

When the members of a family mutually support each other, the burden of the caregiving role is considerably decreased. The quality of care may even be improved if you can gain reassurance from emotional support that a family network can provide. Joint decisions concerning continued care at home or nursing home placement are more easily arrived at when there is less friction and more communication between sisters and brothers, husbands and wives, teenage children and their parents.

A family with a common problem may be drawn closer together by cooperating in the daily care of the chronically ill person and managing his finances and business affairs. Sometimes the reverse happens: families are split apart by jealousy emanating from past experiences, or by misunderstanding the person's condition or what care is essential.

Extended families that become larger because of second marriages may be either a blessing or the source of much conflict. The Riverton family, once a close-knit group, became divided when, Joshua, their 78-year-old father, a widower of four years, married Rosalie, a 72-year-old widow. Both were parents of married children, both lived independently and had their own finances until they met and married in the summer of 1978. The marriage appeared to be successful; they liked each other, Rosalie was a good cook and baker, and Joshua helped her with the shopping and the laundry. They were entertained by their children and friends on birthdays and anniversaries; for Easter and Christmas, they invited everybody to their house and made a big party. It always took them about a week to recover from all the work, but it was worth it, and they were content.

When they had been married about four years, Rosalie noticed that Joshua was starting to forget things and becoming very nasty to her when she mentioned it. This continued to happen for several months. Finally, when Joshua got up one morning and didn't know where he was, she became frightened and called her son. Together they took Joshua to their family physician. The physician, recognizing some of the signs of Alzheimer's disease, suggested that Joshua be sent to a hospital for neurological tests to confirm his diagnosis.

When Joshua was to be released from the hospital, Rosalie refused to take him home. She said she couldn't care for a sick man all by herself. So the social worker called a family conference in order to plan for Joshua's discharge. Both Rosalie's children and Joshua's children were called to the conference. By this time, family hostilities were apparent in the seating arrangements, with the Riverton children seated on one side of the table and the Dinoff family on the other side. They all knew of Rosalie's refusal to take Joshua home. The Riverton children were very angry, and the Dinoff children sided with their mother—after all, she was elderly herself and Joshua had started to become mean to her. They agreed with their mother that Joshua would be too big a burden for her.

The conference included a pyschologist, a social worker, and the head nurse and nurses's aide on the floor. As the psychologist led the discussion, she tried to get each family member's view of the situation. First, they discussed the illness and the fact that it would get progressively worse. Joshua's remaining abilities and what he would have difficulty with were explained by the staff. The group discussed what would have to be done and who could do it; practical issues of daily care and finances for home health aides were brought up, and the possibility of dividing the care among Mr. Riverton's children was bandied about.

The money questions seemed to be a matter of concern. Who would have to pay for this care? Who would inherit the father's money? Did Mr. Riverton make a new will leaving all his assets to Rosalie? Who would pay the bills for the special locks and grab bars that would have to be put into the home of whichever family did take Joshua? Who would be legally responsible for him?

A shrewd woman, Rosalie wanted both sides of the family in on the conference so they would know just what she was up against emotionally, physically, and financially. She knew in advance that she would take Joshua home with her; she loved him and would take care of him as long as she could, but she knew she needed help and wanted that help to come not just from her own children, on whom she knew she could depend, but from Joshua's children also. They were his heirs, so she wanted them to pitch in financially and offer some practical and concrete solutions.

They worked it out that each son and daughter would come one day a week to help Rosalie with whatever shopping needed to be done and with bathing Joshua. This would also give Rosalie some time to herself to go to the beauty parlor and meet her friends once a week for a game of canasta. The grandchildren offered to come and take Grandpa Joshua for a walk on weekends and after school so he could get some exercise. When Rosalie felt satisfied that the responsibilities would be divided among all of the children and that they understood the nature of the illness, she then "changed her mind" and told the staff she would take Joshua home with her.

A week later, Ms. Daly, the social worker, made a home visit to see how Joshua and Rosalie were doing. Rosalie said that so far everyone had lived up to the bargain, and things were going smoothly, so she didn't feel unduly burdened. She felt sad for Joshua, and she and the children were able to talk about how painful it was to see him looking so healthy but obviously confused and not in touch with what was going on around him.

Caregivers need the support of other relatives; they also must have the support and services of friends, neighbors, the community, home attendants and health aides, and whatever hospital or nursing facilities are available for temporary or respite services.

Above all, family members are faced with a mixture of feelings that motivate caregiving behavior. Affection and compassion may motivate devotion to a parent or spouse; but attitudes about duty and responsibility are also reasons for dedication, and these may lead to feelings of resentment and hostility toward a person who is dependent upon you. In turn, you may wish to deny the extent of the person's illness, feel angry about it, become depressed and unable to express the anger and sadness; ultimately you will feel very guilty for having any or all of these feelings.

Sharing your pain, anguish, grief, and angry feelings not only with one another but also with members of other families who are in similar circumstances and who will listen as well as empathize is a unique experience for caregivers. Support groups can fill some of the needs of families that are caring for a person with Alzheimer's disease. In such groups, caregivers also benefit each other by sharing information about managing the patient at home, financial and medical information, and practical guidance about home care.

To the person who gives daily care to someone with Alzheimer's disease, one problem seems to dwarf all the others, and that is loneliness.

Ms. MARGARET ARTHUR: "It's a cross you have to bear, in a way. You don't walk with anybody. You don't talk with anybody. You live with somebody and there's no communication whatsoever. It makes you feel very lonely."

Self-Help Support Groups

Self-help support groups have sprung up through the country among people who share the common burden of caring for a relative with Alzheimer's disease or a similar chronic illness. The Alzheimer's Disease and Related Disorders Association, which has chapters nationwide, has helped many people to organize group meetings where they can come together and discuss their problems and their feelings.

Support groups are exactly that—groups whose major purpose is to encourage families to feel less alone and to help each other. These are nonprofessional groups, primarily volunteer organizations, usually started by family members who recognize their need to share, face to face with other caregivers, the burden of caring for a person with Alzheimer's disease.

Such family support groups offer information about the illness, lists of available resources such as physicians and psychotherapists, and ideas on how to manage the patient at home. They may also relieve the caregiver's sense of isolation and offer friendship. (Contact the national organization or the ADRDA office in the area nearest you for the address of local groups. See Appendix A.)

On occasion, an interested professional counselor, psychotherapist, or gerontologist with counseling skills may attend some sessions, establish discussion groups for family members, or help them to set up their own. Someone with leadership skills, such as a teacher or a clergyman, may be interested in helping to form the group. Members of the group generally assume personal responsibility for organizing the meetings and sharing information. While such groups sometimes offer material assistance, they are mostly for emotional support. Usually groups meet once a week for an hour and a half in someone's home, or in a church or school. Refreshments are served, some agenda for the meeting is specified, and each member of the group expresses his views about the topic. Mutual cooperation is stressed; members are encouraged to listen to each other and offer advice.

MR. BENJAMIN CAREW: "When I first joined the support group, I asked myself, 'Why am I doing this? Why should I come and listen to everyone else's troubles? I've already got enough of my own.' But now I find that I'm benefiting from it. When I walk out of a meeting, I don't feel lost like I did before. I've learned that there are other people in the same position I am in. And besides that, I've spent an hour or two with other people, very pleasantly, listening to adult conversation, which is something I no longer have at home.

"In my support group there are people who really care what I have to say about my brother. When my friends ask me, 'How's your brother?' I always say the same thing: 'Getting along.' That's all I say. What am I going to say? I used to tell them what it was really like, and then I realized they didn't really want to hear the details. They only ask you to be nice. But the people in my support group really listen."

It is important to remember, however, that self-help support groups, while offering support and encouragement, are *not* psychotherapy groups and usually operate without any professional guidance. In a psychotherapy group, feelings may be explored in depth with a skilled psychotherapist who can help the group member not only to verbalize his feelings, as he might in a support group, but also to come to terms with them. By understanding and accepting his feelings, arriving at alternative solutions to the behaviors that these feelings provoke in him, and finding respite from his pain, all of which are possible in a psychotherapy group, the caregiving group member can find relief from depression and return to zestful and joyful living.

Choosing Psychotherapy for the Caregiver

Should you go to a support group, or do you need individual counseling or group psychotherapy?

Most caregivers are so shocked and grieved upon learning that a loved one has Alzheimer's disease that they don't know what to do. They may turn to a friend or neighbor who may not be well informed. Even physicians may not be aware of Alzheimer's support groups for relatives or other resources.

However, there are those caregivers who become very depressed, especially as the burden of caring for the Alzheimer's patient increases over time. These people should seek the help of a psychotherapist who is knowledgeable about treating depression and about the particular stresses that Alzheimer's disease brings to a family. Depression can best be worked through with a skilled professional psychotherapist or psychoanalyst, individually or in a group. A psychotherapist can help caregivers understand the course of Alzheimer's disease, the nature of their own depression (is it chronic or reactive to the circumstances?), how to deal with their feelings, and how to restructure their thinking so that they can mobilize themselves to do what is necessary for their own survival and that of the Alzheimer's victim. It is extremely important to remember that you cannot minister to the needs of another human being if you cannot minister to your own needs first. Nurturing, empathy, and compassion for oneself are the prerequisites for being able to nurture another with love, warmth, compassion, and empathy.

It is not incompatible for a caregiver to go to a support group and also to have individual psychotherapy, but when time and money are important factors (as they often are), it might be wiser to opt for individual treatment first. Once you are feeling more in control of yourself and your life, you will then find attending a support group a more palatable and useful experience.

Mrs. Jay saw her therapist for approximately one year after her beloved and admired husband had been diagnosed as having Alzheimer's disease. She had taken care of him for three years before his diagnosis, catering to his every need, finding things that both of them could do to enjoy a bit of the day. They would walk on the boardwalk or have coffee with some of her friends. But lately Mr. Jay had become restless, easily distracted, harder to manage. Mrs. Jay's friends declined her invitations, and walking became more difficult for Mr. Jay.

Mrs. Jay became very depressed. Sent by her son, himself a therapist, Mrs. Jay and her psychotherapist discussed the anger she felt at her husband, some of which predated his illness. He had been a workaholic, had often come home late, and had had little time or energy for Mrs. Jay. She was remorseful because in her anger she had yelled at her husband and called him names. Her only respite had been seeing her daughter and grandson, but these visits were occasional.

Much of the deep sadness that Mrs. Jay felt was in mourning for the lost affections, sex, and companionship of her husband. She also mourned the loss of the plans they had made for their retirement years, such as traveling together to their native European birthplace.

A very dependent woman, Mrs. Jay had experienced many traumas as a survivor of war and imprisonment. These experiences also contributed to her depression and had to be talked about, emotionally refelt, and worked through before her depression would lift and she would be able to continue to go on caring for her husband. Suicidal thoughts and feelings were part of her depression. She needed the caring and nurturing of a trained psychotherapist to help her recognize she was expecting too much from herself, and to ease her guilt about not being an adequate caregiver to her husband (and to other family members earlier in her life).

After a few months Mrs. Jay began to feel better, look better, and take control of her life. She engaged two home attendants and learned to be able to give herself an hour or two to read, relax, meet with neighbors, and reap some small pleasures from her life. Eventually, as her husband deteriorated, she decided to place him in a nursing home. Although it was a difficult decision, she discussed it with her psychotherapist, expressing her guilty feelings, tracing them back to feelings of guilt about not doing enough for her mother, always needing to be the "good girl" who sacrificed her life for others so they would love her.

Mrs. Jay was *now* ready to join a support group and continue her visits to her husband in the nursing home, as well as to think of some pleasant things she could do in her own life, such as weekending with her daughter or planning a vacation. Without individual psychotherapy she would not have been able to resolve her guilt, work through her depression, and make a life for herself.

A pilot study of counseling for clients with mild Alzheimer's disease, reported in the *Journal of Neurological Rehabilitation* in 1988, revealed that the patients developed helpful attitudes, used coping mechanisms, and identified strategies to compensate for and deal with memory loss. Nevertheless, there were individual differences in receptivity to counseling in the twenty-two patients, who ranged in age from 68 to 84. In other words, this study found that counseling can help some patients more than others.

Individual and Group Psychotherapy

MR. PETER IVORSON: "I met a woman whose brother was even further along in the disease than my dad. And she works full-time, so she has to have full-time help to take care of him. But I don't think she has tried to seek out any support group. When I called her up and told her that there was a group being started in our neighborhood, she was very guarded. I guess it's very hard to admit that your relative has this disease. You know that something's wrong when you don't want to admit that you could use the help."

Mr. Ivorson is perceptive in his appreciation of how painful it is to confront the reality of a relative's disability. Many people, for a variety of reasons, find it difficult to seek the help they need. In particular, for a majority of older people, psychotherapy is still anathema, or, at the very least, looked on with suspicion. They were brought up to be fiercely independent and to keep their thoughts and innermost feelings to themselves, or to share them only with a confidant. The idea of going to a stranger for help is frowned upon; it is considered demeaning and would be humiliating for some. Others have had friends or relatives who have shared their experiences with a psychotherapist and are less afraid to admit their need for help from a professional person.

INDIVIDUAL PSYCHOTHERAPY

When internal conflicts prevent people from being able to work, love, and play effectively, individual psychotherapy can be extremely useful. It helps to resolve worries and fears that may prevent personal and career success. For the person who is caring for a memory-impaired relative and finding the burden nearly insupportable and his emotions running out of control, psychotherapy offers an opportunity for relief through personal change. By uncovering underlying conflicts, discharging and working through anxiety-provoking, hostile, sexual, and dependency feelings, you will find different and creative options for dealing with internal stress and stressful life situations. Your curiosity will be kept alive, for you will not turn your back on yourself or on life.

GROUP PSYCHOTHERAPY

Relatives whose memory-impaired patients live at home often find it extremely useful and helpful to become part of a supportive psychotherapy group. Members of the group understand your situation and can be empathic to your feelings. Often the group, or the leader of the group (who is a skilled and qualified group psychotherapist) will be able to help you recognize that you are depressed. The psychotherapist helps you to work through your depressed feelings and your daily suffering will be reduced.

Family members who share the problems of living with an impaired relative can, in group therapy, learn how to get along better with each other and how to improve their patterns of interaction with the memory-impaired patient. They learn to understand their own feelings of guilt, anger, resentment, anxiety, and frustration and develop techniques to deal with these feelings. Practical skills and guides to managing the behavior of the Alzheimer's patient at home are also learned. Discussions about preparing for the possibility that they will have to place an Alzheimer's patient in an institution are considered from the point of view that placement may become a desirable alternative to continued home care, when home care becomes too difficult or exhausting.

Finally, they may develop a more accepting attitude, both toward their patient and toward themselves. When family caregivers feel emotionally supported as they do in a group therapy setting, they may be saved from feelings of despair and anguish.

MR. WILLARD RAEBURN: "Your spirits are lifted when you can talk about your problems in a group that understands. I don't know where else you could talk about it.

"People avoid the subject. There's no way to talk about it unless you just plunge in and say, 'Why don't you talk to me about my wife?' And you can't do that. I don't want to do that. I need to feel that they're

329

interested in me, in my problem, and not just that I'm pouring it on until I bore them to death.

"Going to my group has helped to lessen that feeling of isolation. I find a response there from people who really understand, because they're sharing the same problems."

In the group, you and other caregivers can recognize and assess your strengths as well as your weaknesses. You will begin to see yourself in relation to others, and you won't feel quite so alone. You can grow emotionally by learning to take support from the other members in the group and to give support in return.

The most powerful message that most caregivers receive upon first joining a group is that feelings of shame, humiliation, anger, guilt, and depression are normal under the stresses of loss. Many people describe the feeling of loss with the statement "It feels like the rug has been pulled out from under me." The feelings of helplessness and hopelessness that plague us when the people we've depended upon are no longer available to us can be ameliorated by sharing them with the group. The psychotherapy group enables you to feel that you can go on—and indeed you must.

Group psychotherapy promotes personal growth through sharing feelings, ideas, and emotional difficulties with others. The psychotherapist and other group members may be able to hear your innermost thoughts and feelings, which alone you fail to recognize or acknowledge. The group also offers moral support, objective criticism, and useful suggestions for alternative ways of coping with life. Deep social responses are activated through identifying with other people's pain and understanding their dilemmas.

How You and Your Psychotherapist Can Work Together

The relationship with your psychotherapist, either in individual or group psychotherapy, is a most crucial factor in the successful treatment of all patients, including the elderly. Many therapists will be younger than their patients; it is natural to feel some resentment because of this, and it is important that you share this feeling with the therapist.

Your therapy will be extremely valuable to you if you can conceive of it as a joint exploration embarked on by you and your therapist. Through a review of your life and reminiscences about the losses you anticipate or have experienced, you will be able to express your feelings about these losses and what they have meant to you. You will unlearn those behaviors and attitudes that have caused you pain, and then relearn new, more positive ways to meet your own needs. By providing opportunities for you to rid yourself of anger, guilt, and other painful feelings, as well as attitudes and thoughts that interfere with your ability to think and feel more positively and lovingly, therapy will help you feel less alone and more in touch with the world.

An empathic therapist will understand your feelings and provide an environment in which corrective experiences and taking risks can be discussed and dramatically enacted. The confidentiality of your psychotherapy sessions, whether individual or group, will help you to discuss things that make you feel ashamed and embarrassed or fearful.

In time, you will develop trust and confidence in your therapist; however, there may be moments when you will feel reluctant to tell your therapist everything that is on your mind, especially if there is something about the therapy or the therapist that displeases you. Remember that the first rule of therapy is to divulge all. Your ability to ventilate your grievances and resentments will help you to dissipate the guilt you feel. If you feel too dependent on the therapist, it is important to remember that this is part of the therapy process and is helpful in allowing you to feel safe and cared about.

Eventually, when your therapy is concluded, there will be separation from the therapist. You may find that you have mixed (positive and negative) feelings at that point; these feelings occur in every relationship where one person feels dependent on another. Working through the ambivalence, which means recognizing the privileges and also the responsibilities of every relationship, helps to put the relationship in perspective.

Neither the therapist nor anyone in your past or present life can fulfill all your unrealized pleasures, or make up for all the deprivations in the past. It is regrettable but inevitable that not all of our needs, wishes, fantasies, or dreams have been fulfilled by parents, spouse, children, teachers, therapists, or any godlike figures that we have imbued with such powers. Understanding this helps us to relinquish the desire for perfection in others and in ourselves. The knowledge that they did their best for us is sufficient. Now it is up to us to have the courage to do the best we can with whatever love, talents, abilities, beauty, money, skills, or time that we have left.

Most reputable and skilled psychotherapists do not have a vested interest in keeping you as a patient beyond the time it takes for you to accomplish your goals. There are, however, as in every group, some "bad apples" who do prolong treatment to enrich themselves. If you have doubts about the necessity of further treatment, discuss these doubts with your therapist, and if you are not satisfied, seek a consultation with another psychotherapist. Always look up your psychotherapist in a local or national directory to assure yourself that the psychotherapist has the appropriate education and credentials. Discuss the therapist's credentials in the first visit, along with the fee, the length and frequency of sessions, and the issue of confidentiality. (Two directories you may want to use are those of the American Psychological Association and the National Association for the Advancement of Psychoanalysis.)

We hope that the next generation of older people will be more familiar with the various types of psychotherapy available, including individual, group, family, or marital therapy. Our hope is that they will value psychotherapy as a tool to facilitate emotional health and will pursue it as readily as they seek medical attention when necessary.

Periodic preventive emotional health checkups are now being subscribed to by those advocates of psychotherapy who are familiar with the process and aware of its potential for sustaining emotional health and a state of emotional well-being.

In support and therapy groups, caregivers share their loneliness with one another. They exchange their stories, loving and humorous, painful and exasperating; they share their feelings about smashed hopes and disappointments and loving anecdotes that are all part of their burden of love. Even those who have, however reluctantly, placed their impaired relatives in nursing homes discover that wherever their patient is, he remains central in the hearts and minds of those who have suffered through this illness with him.

Yet, whatever the connections to the Alzheimer's patient appear to be, in truth, each one of us remains alone. It is an unalterable fact of life. We are all existentially alone, and we must learn to accept the realization that, just as the birth process was a solitary experience, so will be our passage from life to death. Once we can understand and accept that this is the nature of life, life itself becomes less fearful and traumatic.

Our feelings of loneliness can be lived through. We can accept the understanding that the essence of life is change, and that growth and renewal are as possible as loss and despair.

Ms. Susan Harness: "I'll never forget the last Christmas that my father was alive. We had finally put him in the nursing home, just a week or two before, because he had become so confused that he was wandering day and night and was very abusive to Mom. He was not physically well, so we all came home, gloomily, thinking it was going to be a dreadful time. But my sister brought her little three-month-old baby. That child was so full of sunshine! All of us were aware of the ebullience of life in that baby, and I think it made the realization of my father's impending death somehow easier to accept."

Having accepted our feelings of loneliness and loss, we no longer feel devastated and are ready to make the next move to soothing ourselves, taking comfort and solace in the pleasures and gifts of life that enrich the human spirit. But we must be prepared for new adventures by allowing ourselves to partake of them. We've earned them. The best in life may still be yet to come.

Friends can help. When they call and say, "Come with us," don't hesitate to go; share some pleasant moments with them.

Ms. JENNIFER ANDERS: "My sister is very nice to us, and her husband is wonderful! Every Saturday, they call us in the morning and ask, 'What are you doing today?' (What am I doing today? What am I always doing? I tell people I feel like I spend my life serving soup with a strainer.) 'Would you like to go to lunch with us?' they ask.

"We go to a nearby diner or fast-food place. My husband gets along better with my brother-in-law then he does with his own brother. He'll sit there in the restaurant for an hour or more, making garbled sounds with an occasional recognizable word or two, nothing coherent, and my brother-in-law listens to him.

"And that's all. Then we'll go home and he'll say 'Thank you.' Soon he goes to sleep.

"For myself, I enjoy having the opportunity for some intelligent conversation and being with my sister and her husband for the hour or two that we're at lunch."

To find ways to relieve your loneliness and share your life with others, use your imagination, just as you did when your children were small and you found ways to join with other parents to do the things you wanted for yourself and your children. Learn what services are available in your apartment building, on your block, or around the corner, if you live in the city. In the suburbs, find out about car pools and special services provided by the county and your Chamber of Commerce and the local Department of Aging. If none are available, start you own support or interest group. Put up notices at the local supermarket, or run an ad in the local newspaper.

How Some Caregivers Reshape Their Lives

We are not going to tell you that changing your focus in this way is a simple task. It requires strength, an acceptance of your own feelings, and sometimes the help and intervention of a counselor as well. Harry Atkins is a still-youthful man in his early sixties. He has lived through three years of painful changes in his beloved wife, Geraldine, who developed Alzheimer's disease while in her fifties and declined rapidly. Mr. Atkins dragged his wife from one doctor to another, put her in and out of research programs, and tried all types of medications in a futile effort to cure her. Finally, when Geraldine tried to stab him with a butcher knife in one of her frequent violent outbursts, he decided to commit her to the state hospital. An adoring husband, he visited her at the hospital almost daily until a psychiatrist told him to do himself a favor, cut his visits to once a week, and stop neglecting himself.

Geraldine's devoted cousin, Kathleen, quickly became a source of great comfort to Mr. Atkins:

> "Lately, I've been seeing a lot of Kathleen, Geraldine's third cousin by marriage—she's good company. We've all been friends for years. I knew her parents and used to tease her when she was growing up. But at this point, I'm so depressed that I can't even enjoy her company. We go out; she even comes to visit Geraldine with me. Kathleen's a fine, independent woman—a widow—has grown children, a house, and lots of guts. It's comforting to have a companion to talk to and someone to laugh with, but sexually—no way . . . I can't do it. What's wrong with me?"

Mr. Atkins feels very guilty about "dumping" Geraldine. While he and Kathleen like each other, and find themselves physically attracted to one another, Mr. Atkins's feeling that he has betrayed Geraldine with Kathleen probably contributes to his psychologically induced impotence. On the other hand, he feels he can't offer marriage to Kathleen, and so he also feels guilty about that. Moreover, he is financially responsible for Geraldine's care, whether she remains in the state institution or goes to a nursing home, but the difference in cost is practically one-third. That also worries Mr. Atkins; he's afraid he will have to mortgage his business to pay for his wife's care.

Mr. Atkins has been depressed for a year, although he has only become aware of how bad he feels in the last six months, since institutionalizing his wife.

Under the circumstances, Mr. Atkins is very angry at himself. He is also angry at his wife for becoming ill, and "betraying" their forty-year marriage. "It was supposed to be 'till death do us part,' but even though the wedding vows also include 'in sickness and in health,' who ever dreamed that we'd wind up this way? It's a living hell!"

Mr. Atkins's story is one of many. He is among those who call themselves the "married widows and widowers." These caregivers face the predicament of still being physically and emotionally wed to their impaired and often unresponsive spouses, while at the same time needing and desiring companionship, sexual fulfillment, and a loving relationship with someone who can return the feeling. Still tied to the memories of the lives they shared with the victims of Alzheimer's disease, they face the necessity of "starting over," meeting new people, going out, dating, and trying to find a compatible friend who will share, or at least understand, the dilemma in which they find themselves.

The guilt of having placed an impaired spouse in a nursing home is great; the even greater guilt of betraying the spouse with another person haunts the new relationship and can indeed lead to psychological symptoms such as impotence and depression. For you, the caregiving spouse who has not been the unfortunate victim of Alzheimer's disease, guilt may be standing in the way of your finding the will to go on and to enjoy life once again. In psychotherapy, guilt can be talked about and worked through so that some fairly normal relationships can ensue.

Learning to live alone after years of living with someone can be as frightening to an older person as it can be to the young adult who goes out on his own for the first time. For many older people, this will be the first time they have been alone since leaving the home of their parents. It takes a period of adjustment to learn to take care of yourself and to give yourself the things you need to help make being alone more of an adventure than a prison sentence. Some people find they simply are not comfortable living alone and will choose companions. Others will be content to be on their own and not seek a relationship other than the comfort of friends, family, and pets.

Ilona Swenson had to start from scratch after she placed her 70-year-old husband, Per, in a nursing home. Having had emergency kidney surgery at the same time as her husband was admitted to the home, Ilona hadn't seen Per for about four months. When she was well enough to visit, although she didn't know what to expect when she got there, she made the trip to the nursing home with her daughter Jill and her son-in-law. Jill and her husband had both prepared Ilona for the fact that Per might not recognize her.

When they arrived at the home, Ilona steeled herself and cautiously but eagerly walked toward Per. He was sitting in a wheelchair, staring vacantly ahead, but as she approached, he began a smile that spread from ear to ear.

"Do you know who that is?" asked Jill.

"Ilona," he answered, and as he beamed, tears fell from his eyes. They were both overjoyed to be reunited, and parting was difficult. "He wanted to go home with me," Ilona recalled when she described the scene. "But I told him I'd be back soon. The nurses told me not to worry, that they would take care of him. They were accustomed to the problem and knew how to handle it."

A few days later, Jill asked her mother how she would feel about seeing other men. To her surprise, Ilona said, "Well, he'd have to be a very special man, not just anybody." Still pretty and youthful at 65, Ilona had thought about her years with Per—they were good, productive, joyful years. She also thought about being alone for the rest of her life, and although she would be devoted to Per until his very last breath, she would welcome some congenial male companionship. A practical woman who loves to go to the theater and to dance, Ilona is readying herself physically and psychologically to meet someone to become a friend and perhaps a lover.

But first, before other relationships can become important, the primary relationship with the living, albeit impaired, spouse must be put into perspective and mourned. Then the guilt must be worked through, in order to make it possible for new feelings to develop—new feelings for another person that could ease the loneliness and enrich the years to come with new experiences.

Epilogue

Alzheimer's disease is a burden that only the patient can forget. We are all victims of this tragic illness. Only through public recognition of the enormity of the problem of Alzheimer's disease and its emotional and economic impact on the family and on society will new funding and adequate resources become a government priority. We should educate our legislators and alert them to the fact that about two million people suffer impairment through some form of memory loss and two million more suffer from mild cognitive impairment.

All too often, legislators and professional people only take notice of the severity of the illness when one of their own family members becomes afflicted. You can be instrumental in bringing this dread disease out into public awareness by educating yourself, your family, neighbors, and friends. Talk to people. Write your concerns to the National Council on Aging and to your state and local aging offices. Work with organizations for advocacy for the elderly. Get the press interested in these issues.

Whatever you have gained from reading this book, share it, not only with people who are personally involved with a memory-impaired relative, but also with others who may benefit. Remember these helpful words:

- Take life one day at a time.
- Know your limitations.
- Acknowledge that your supreme value is love.
- Send your love out into the world—it will flow back to you.
- Be positive about life, laugh, and discover joy in living.

If just one person benefits from having read this book, we will have accomplished our goal.

339

Resources

Alzheimer's Disease and
Related Disorders
919 N. Michigan Ave.
Suite 100
Chicago, IL 60611
(800) 272-3900

Alzheimer's Disease and
Related Disorders
(International Association)
919 N. Michigan Ave.
Suite 100
Chicago, IL 60611
Contact: Rachel Billington
(312) 335-8700, x3777

Alzheimer's Society for
Metropolitan Toronto
980 Young St.
Suite 301
Toronto, Ontario M4W 2J5
Canada
(416) 966-0700

Alzheimer's Society of Canada
1200 Bay St.
Suite 202
Toronto, Ontario M5R 2A5
Canada
(416) 967-5900

American Association of Homes
for the Aging
901 E St. NW
Suite 500
Washington, DC 20004
(202) 783-2242

American Health Assistance Foundation
15825 Shady Grove Rd.
Suite 140
Rockville, MD 20850
(301) 948-3244
Publishes *Alzheimer's Research Review*, a
quarterly newsletter summarizing the
work of Alzheimer's disease researchers.

Choice In Dying
200 Varick St.
New York, NY 10014
(212) 366–5540

Family Service America
11700 W. Lake Park Dr.
Milwaukee, Wisconsin 53224
(414) 359–1040

Friends and Relatives of
Institutionalized Aged
11 John St.
New York, NY 10038
(212) 732–4455

Family Survival Program for Brain-
Damaged Adults
425 Bush St.
Suite 500
San Francisco, CA 94108
(415) 434–3388

Gerontological Society
1275 K St. NW
Suite 350
Washington, DC 20005–4006
(202) 842–1275

Hemlock Society of Los Angeles
P.O. Box 60218
Los Angeles, CA 90066
(310) 476–8696

Medic Alert International
Turlock, CA 95380
(209) 632–2371

National Association for Home Care
519 C St. NE
Washington, DC 20002
(202) 547–7424

Partners in Care
5 Penn Plaza
18th Floor
New York, NY 10001
(212) 330–7700

In addition to these national organizations, there are many resources available to you locally. Find the visiting nurses association in your phone book. The state or city government probably has offices dealing with nursing homes and perhaps even with the specific needs of people with Alzheimer's disease; again, consult your local phone directory.

Resident's Bill of Rights

The resident's rights policies and procedures shall ensure that, at least, each resident admitted:[1]

is fully informed, as evidenced by the resident's written acknowledgment, prior to or at the time of admission and during stay, of these rights and is given a statement of the facility's rules and regulations, and an explanation of the resident's responsibility to obey all reasonable regulations of the facility and to respect the personal rights and private property of other residents;

is fully informed, and is given a written statement prior to or at the time of admission and during stay, of services available in the facility, and of related charges including any charges for services not covered by sources of third-party payments or not covered by the facility's basic per diem rate;

is assured of adequate and appropriate medical care, is fully informed, by a physician, of his medical condition unless medically contraindicated (as documented, by a physician, in his medical record), is afforded the opportunity to participate in the planning of his medical treatment, to

1. Abstracted from 1CNYCRR Chapter 5 of the State Hospital Code; applies to nursing homes and health-related facilities.

refuse to participate in experimental research, and to refuse medication and treatment after being fully informed of and understanding the consequences of such actions;

is transferred or discharged only for medical reasons, or for his welfare or that of other residents, or for nonpayment for his stay (except as prohibited by sources of third-party payment), and is given reasonable advance notice to ensure orderly transfer or discharge, and such actions are documented in his medical record;

is encouraged and assisted, throughout his period of stay, to exercise his rights as a resident and as a citizen, and to this end may voice grievances, has a right of action for damages or other relief for deprivations or infringements of his right to adequate and proper treatment and care established by any applicable statute, rule, regulation, or contract, and to recommend changes in policies and services to facility staff and/or to outside representatives of his choice, free from restraint, interference, coercion, discrimination, or reprisal;

may manage his personal financial affairs, or is given at least a quarterly accounting of financial transactions made on his behalf should the facility accept his written delegation of this responsibility to the facility for any period of time in conformance with state law;

is free from mental and physical abuse, and free from chemical and physical restraints except those restraints authorized in writing by a physician for a specified and limited period of time or when necessary to protect the resident from injury to himself or to others, or as are necessitated by an emergency, in which case the restraint may only be applied by a licensed nurse who shall set forth in writing the circumstances requiring the use of restraint; in the case of use of a chemical restraint, a physician shall be consulted within 24 hours;

is assured security in storing personal possessions and confidential treatment of his personal and medical records, and may approve or refuse their release to any individual outside the facility, except in the case of his transfer to another health-care institution, or as required by law or third-party payment contract;

is treated with consideration, respect, and full recognition of his dignity and individuality, including privacy in treatment and in care for his personal needs;

is not required to perform services for the facility that are not included for therapeutic purposes in his plan of care;

may associate and communicate privately with persons of his choice, may join with other residents or individuals within or outside of the facility to work for improvements in resident care, and send and receive his personal mail unopened, unless medically contraindicated (as documented by his physician in his medical record);

may meet with, and participate in activities of social, religious, and community groups at his discretion, unless medically contraindicated (as documented by his physician in his medical record);

may retain and use his personal clothing and possessions as space permits, unless to do so would infringe upon rights of other residents, unless medically contraindicated (as documented by his physician in his medical record);

if married, is assured privacy for visits by his/her spouse; if both are residents in the facility, they are permitted to share a room, unless medically contraindicated (as documented by the attending physician in the medical record); and

is assured of exercising his civil and religious liberties, including the right to independent personal decisions, and knowledge of available choices shall not be infringed and the facility shall encourage and assist in the fullest possible exercise of these rights.

Living Wills

A living will is a declaration that the signer does not want certain extraordinary medical procedures used to preserve his life if he is terminally ill. In addition, a patient may appoint another person to make decisions as his health-care agent if he can no longer do so himself.

Because the requirements for a valid living will vary from state to state, the document that follows is just an example. As of May 1992 only three states do not allow living wills, although they do recognize health-care agents: Massachusetts, Michigan, and New York. It is valuable to have a living will even if your state would not recognize it now because the laws may change. The Choice In Dying organization distributes documents appropriate for each state to its members; contact them at the address listed in Appendix A.

Declaration made this _____ day of _____.
(month, year)
I, _____, being of sound mind, willfully and voluntarily making known my desire that my dying shall not be artificially prolonged under the circumstances set forth below, do hereby declare:

If at any time I should have an incurable injury, disease, or illness regarded as a terminal condition by my physician and if my physician has determined that the application of life-sustaining procedures would serve only to artificially prolong the dying process and that my death will occur whether or not life-sustaining procedures are utilized, I direct that such procedures be withheld or withdrawn and that I be permitted to die with only the administration of medication or the performance of any medical procedure deemed necessary to provide me with comfort care.

In the absence of my ability to give directions regarding the use of such life-sustaining procedures, it is my intention that this declaration shall be honored by my family and physician as the final expression of my legal right to refuse medical or surgical treatment and accept the consequences from such refusal.

I understand the full import of this declaration and I am emotionally and mentally competent to make this declaration.

Signed _____

City, County, and State of Residence _____

The declarant has been personally known to me and I believe him or her to be of sound mind.

Witness _____

Address _____

Witness _____

Address _____

_____
Notary Public

Selected References

Allen, Robert F., with Shirley Linde. *Lifegain*. New York: Appleton-Century-Crofts, 1981.

Alpaugh, P., and M. Haney. *Counseling the Older Adult—A Training Manual for Para-Professionals and Beginning Counselors*. Ethel Percy Andrus Gerontology Center. Los Angeles: University of Southern California Press, 1978.

Alzheimer's Research Review (Spring 1991).

Berezin, M. A., and S. H. Cath. "Grief, Loss, and Emotional Disorders in the Aging Process." In *Geriatric Psychiatry*. New York: International Universities Press, 1965.

Berger, Eugene V. "A System for Rating the Severity of Senility." *Journal of the American Geriatrics Society* 27, no. 5 (1980): 234–36.

Bernheim, Kayla F., et al. *The Caring Family—Living with Chronic Mental Illness*. New York: Random House, 1982.

Blumenthal, M. "Psychosocial Factors in Reversible and Irreversible Brain Failure." *Journal of Clinical Experimental Gerontology* 1 (1979): 39–55.

Bowlby, John. "Attachment and Loss." *Loss, Sadness, and Depression*, vol. 3. New York: Basic Books, Harper & Row, 1980.

The Brain: Mystery of Matter and Mind. Washington, D.C.: U.S. News Books, 1981.

Brody, Jane. *Jane Brody's Nutrition Book—A Lifetime Guide to Good Eating for Better Health and Weight Control*. New York: W. W. Norton and Co., 1981.

Burgalassi, Anthony J. *Living Wills—The Right to Die: A Selective Bibliography with Statutory Appendix*. New York: Martindale-Hubbell Law Digest, 1990.

Burke Rehabilitation Center. "Managing the Person with Intellectual Loss at Home." White Plains, N.Y. 1980.

Butler, R. N., and M. I. Lewis. "Organic Brain Disorders." In *Aging and Mental Health*, 68–82. St. Louis: C. V. Mosby Co., 1973.

Cammer, Leonard, M.D. *Up from Depression*. New York: Pocket Books, Simon & Schuster, 1979.

Choice In Dying, T. Patrick Hill, and David Shirley. *A Good Death: Taking More Control at the End of Your Life*. Reading, Mass.: Addison-Wesley/Lawrence, 1992.

Colbin, Annemarie. *Food and Healing*. New York: Ballantine Books, 1986.

———. *The Natural Gourmet*. New York: Ballantine Books, 1989.

Crook, Thomas, Ph.D., and Samuel Gershon, M.D., eds. *Strategies for the Development of an Effective Treatment for Senile Dementia*. New Canaan, Ct.: Mark Powley Associates, 1981.

Demkovich, Linda E. "In Treating the Problems of the Elderly There May Be No Place Like Home." *National Journal* (December 22, 1979).

Eisdorfer, Carl, Ph.D., and Donna Cohen, Ph.D. "Management of the Patient and Family Coping with Dementing Illness." *Journal of Family Practice* 12, no. 5 (1981): 831–37.

Estella, Mary. *The Natural Foods Cookbook*. New York: Japan Publications, 1985.

Fogelman, E., and B. Savram. "Brief Group Therapy with Offspring of Holocaust Survivors: Leaders' Reactions." *American Journal of Orthopsychiatry* 50, no. 1 (January 1980).

Folstein, M., et al. "Mood Disorder as a Specific Complication of Stroke." *Journal of Neurology, Neurosurgery, and Psychiatry* 40 (1977): 1018–20.

Freyberg, J. T. "Difficulties in Separation—Individuation as Experienced by Offspring of Nazi Holocaust Survivors." *American Journal of Orthopsychiatry* 51, no. 1 (January 1981).

Gautrin, Denyse; Sorona Frode; Hughes Tetrault; et al. (University of Quebec INRS, Sante, Montreal). "Canadian Projection of Cases Suffering from Alzheimer's Disease and Senile Dementia of Alzheimer's Type over Period 1986–2031." *Canadian Journal of Psychology* 35, no. 2 (March 1990).

Gaylin, Willard. *Caring*. New York: Knopf, 1976.

———. *Feelings—Our Vital Signs*. New York: Harper & Row, 1979.

Gianotti, G. "Emotional Behavior and Hemispheric Side of Lesion." *Cortex* 8: 41–55.

Gilhooly, Mary L. M.; Steven Zout; and James Birren, eds. *The Dementias—Policy and Management*. Englewood Cliffs, N.J.: Prentice-Hall, 1986.

Goldberg, Arnold, ed. *Advances in Self-Psychology*. New York: International Universities Press, 1980.

Goldberg, Carl. *Understanding Shame*. Northvale, N.J.: Jason Aronson, 1991.

Goldberg, Z., et al. *The Wadsworth Memory Enhancement Program for Older Adults*. Los Angeles: Neurology Service, V. A. Wadsworth Medical Center, 1980.

Harvard Health Letter 16, no. 9 (July 1991).

Health Insurance News (AARP) 8, no. 1 (Winter 1991).

Henig, Robin Marantz. *The Myth of Senility*. New York: Anchor Press, Doubleday, 1981.

Hinsie, L. E. and R. J. Campbell. *Psychiatric Dictionary*. New York: Oxford University Press, 1980.

Inlander, Charles B., and Charles K. MacKay. *Medicare Made Easy*. Reading, Mass.: Addison-Wesley, 1988.

Institute on Law and Rights of Older Adults. *The Medicaid Program*. New York: Brookdale Center on Aging, Hunter College, 1981.

Justice, Dr. Blair, and Dr. Rita Justice. *The Abusing Family*. New York: Human Sciences Press, 1976.

Keane, Evelyn E., ed. *Coping with Senility: A Guidebook*. Philadelphia: Chronic Organic Brain Syndrome Society, Inc., of Pennsylvania, 1980.

Klein, Melanie, and Joan Riviere. *Love, Hate, and Reparation*. New York: W. W. Norton and Co., 1964.

LaBarge, Emily; Luda S. Rosenna; Katherine Leavitt; and Terese Crishani (Washington University School of Medicine, St. Louis, Mo.). "Counseling Clients with Mild Senile Dementia of the Alzheimer's Disease Type—A Pilot Study." *Journal of Neurologic Rehabilitation* 2, no. 4 (1988): 167–73.

LeRoux, Charles. "The Silent Epidemic." *The Chicago Tribune*, September 1981.

Lazarus, L. W., et al. "A Pilot Study of an Alzheimer Patient's Relatives Discussion Group." *The Gerontologist* 21, no. 4: 353–57.

Mace, Nancy L., and Peter V. Rabins, M.D. *The 36-Hour Day—A Family Guide to Caring for Persons with Alzheimer's Disease, Relating Dementing Illness and Memory Loss in Later Life.* Baltimore: Johns Hopkins University Press, 1981.

Massachusetts General Hospital Newsletter ("Topics in Geriatrics") 1, no. 1 (May 1982).

Miller, Alice. *Prisoners of Childhood.* New York: Basic Books, Inc., Harper & Row, 1982.

Miller, Susan. *The Shame Experience.* New York: Analytic Press, Lawrence Edelbaum Assoc., 1985.

New York Neuropsychology Group Newsletter 1, no. 1 (May 1982).

Nutrition Action Healthletter. "Food Guide Pyramid: A Guide to Daily Food Choice." Washington, D.C.: Center for Science in the Public Interest, July/August 1992.

Parker, C. M. *Bereavement: Studies of Grief in Adult Life.* London: Tavistock Institute of Human Relations, 1972.

Pepper, Claude. "Life in America: Will There Be a Brighter Tomorrow for the Nation's Elderly?" *USA Today*, May 12, 1980.

Powell, Lenore, Ed.D. "Time-Limited Counseling and the Adjustment of New Admissions to Nursing Homes." In *Aging, Isolation, and Resocialization.* Edited by Ruth Bennet. New York: Van Nostrand-Reinhold Co., 1980.

———. "Alzheimer's: The Disease Only the Patient Can Forget." *The Office Nurse* (December 1988).

———. "Be Your Own Nurturer." *The Office Nurse* (May–June 1989).

———. "How to Be Your Own Mother: A Guide to Creative Self-Nurturance." Forthcoming.

Prudden, Bonnie. *Keep Fit, Be Happy.* New York: Warner Bros. Records, Inc. (B-1358), 1960.

Reisberg, Barry, M.D. *Brain Failure.* New York: Free Press, 1981.

Relman, Arnold S. "Special Report: Tacrine as a Treatment for Alzheimer's Disease." *New England Journal of Medicine* (January 31, 1991): 347–52.

Rosenbaum, M., and M. Berger. "A Review of Some Recent Group Psychotherapy Methods for Elderly Psychiatric Patients." In *Group Psychotherapy and Group Function*, 445–95. New York: Basic Books, Harper & Row, 1963.

Schulz, R. *The Psychology of Death, Dying, and Bereavement.* Reading, Mass., Addison-Wesley, 1978.

Selye, Hans. *Stress without Distress.* New York: New American Library, 1974.

Sheikle, Anees. "Picture of Health." *Omni* (February 1989): 105–10.

Silverstone, Barbara, and Helen Kandel Hyman. *You and Your Aging Parent.* New York: Pantheon Books, Random House, 1976.

Solkoff, N. "Children of Survivors of Nazi Holocaust: A Critical Review of the Literature." *American Journal of Orthopsychiatry* 51, no. 1 (January 1981).

Stedman's Medical Dictionary. 22d ed. Baltimore: The Williams & Wilkins Co., 1972.

United States Pharmacopeial Convention, Inc. *The Physicians' and Pharmacists' Guide to Your Medicines.* New York: Ballantine Books, 1981.

Weiner, Marcella B., Ed.D., and Marjorie T. White, Ph.D. "Depression as the Search for the Lost Self." *Psychotherapy: Theory, Research, and Practice* 19, no. 4 (Winter 1982): 491–99.

Weiner, Marcella B., Ed.D.; A. J. Brok; and A. M. Snadowsky. *Working with the Aged.* Englewood Cliffs, N.J.: Prentice-Hall, 1978.

Weinstein, Pearl. "Stroke and Depression: My Father's Case." *New York Neuropsychology Group Newsletter* 1, no. 1 (May 1982).

Wellness Today: A Special Supplement to Health and Healing. Potomac, Md.: Phillips Publishing, May 1992.

Wikler, L., et al. "Chronic Sorrow Revisited: Parents vs. Professional Depiction of the Adjustment of Parents of Mentally Retarded Children." *American Journal of Orthopsychiatry* 51, no. 1 (January 1981).

Williams, Marilyn P. "Alzheimer's Unit by Design." *Geriatric Nursing* (January–February 1991): 34–36.

Winograd, Elliot C., Esq. "The Right to Die: A Review of the Current Status of New York Law: The Derivation of the Principles and the Ethical Considerations." *Trial Lawyers Quarterly* 20, no. 1 (1991).

Yalom, I. D. *The Theory and Practice of Group Psychotherapy,* 2d ed. New York: Basic Books, Harper & Row, 1975.

Index